Nina Hartley's

Guide to TOTAL SEX

Nina Hartley's

Guide to TOTAL

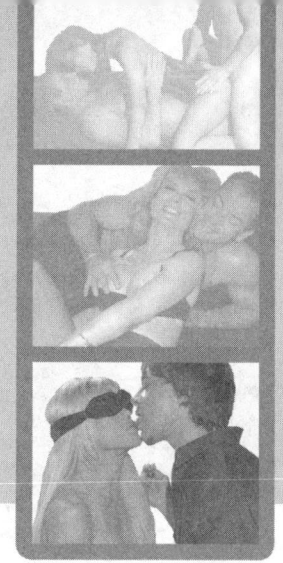

SEX

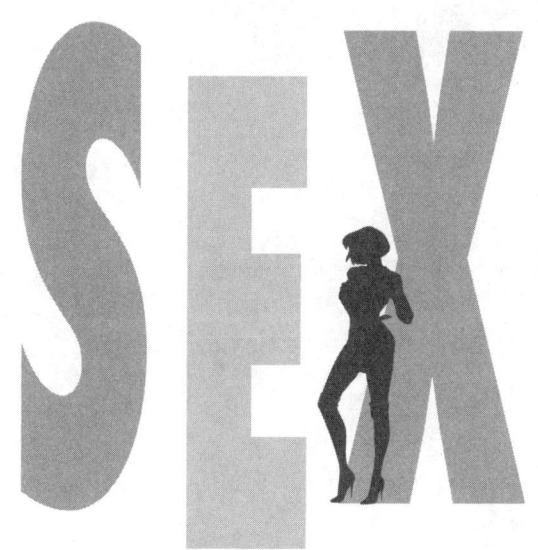

NINA HARTLEY

with I. S. Levine

AVERY
A MEMBER OF
PENGUIN GROUP (USA) INC.
NEW YORK

AVERY

Published by the Penguin Group

Penguin Group (USA) Inc., 375 Hudson Street, New York, New York 10014, USA • Penguin Group (Canada),
90 Eglinton Avenue East, Suite 700, Toronto, Ontario M4P 2Y3, Canada (a division of Pearson Penguin Canada Inc.) •
Penguin Books Ltd, 80 Strand, London WC2R 0RL, England • Penguin Ireland, 25 St Stephen's Green, Dublin 2, Ireland
(a division of Penguin Books Ltd) • Penguin Group (Australia), 250 Camberwell Road, Camberwell, Victoria 3124, Australia
(a division of Pearson Australia Group Pty Ltd) • Penguin Books India Pvt Ltd, 11 Community Centre, Panchsheel Park,
New Delhi–110 017, India • Penguin Group (NZ), Cnr Airborne and Rosedale Roads, Albany, Auckland 1310, New Zealand
(a division of Pearson New Zealand Ltd) • Penguin Books (South Africa) (Pty) Ltd, 24 Sturdee Avenue, Rosebank,
Johannesburg 2196, South Africa

Penguin Books Ltd, Registered Offices: 80 Strand, London WC2R 0RL, England

Photos courtesy Adam&Eve, taken by Vic Alpine

Most Avery books are available at special quantity discounts for bulk purchase for sales promotions, premiums, fund-raising, and educational needs. Special books or book excerpts also can be created to fit specific needs. For details, write Penguin Group (USA) Inc.
Special Markets, 375 Hudson Street, New York, NY 10014.

Library of Congress Cataloging-in-Publication Data

Hartley, Nina.
[Guide to total sex]
Nina Hartley's guide to total sex/by Nina Hartley with I. S. Levine.
p.   cm.
ISBN 1-58333-263-4
1. Sex instruction.   2. Sex.   3. Sexual excitement.   I. Levine, I. S. (Ira S.), 1952–   II. Title.
III. Title: Guide to total sex.
HQ31.H355   2006   2006042966
619'.6—dc22

Printed in the United States of America
3   5   7   9   10   8   6   4

This book is printed on acid-free paper. ♾

BOOK DESIGN BY TANYA MAIBORODA

For Dr. Betty A. Dodson,
who set it all in motion

ACKNOWLEDGMENTS

I would like to give thanks to the many people who helped me so much in the making of this book: Dr. Carol Queen; Dr. Robert Lawrence; Dr. Annie Sprinkle; Patrick Califia, MFCC; Timothy Greenfield-Sanders; Scott Waxman; Farley Chase; Phil Harvey; Bernard Oakley; Bob Christian; Zoe Diamassis; Frank Gavin; Nadine Strossen; Professor Linda Williams; Lou and Blanche Hartman; Joseph Levine; Matthew Brand; Benjamin Hoffman; Jennifer Ramsey; Michelle Beacham; Joel Berens; Olivia De Berardinis; and Veronica Rush. Many thanks to Adam&Eve for the use of their photographs and to the performers whose likenesses illuminate these pages: Shayla Laveaux; Carmen Luvana; Violet Blue; T. J. Hart; Nicole Sheriden; Randy Spears; Christian; Chris Cannon; Voodoo, Trent Tesaro, and Julian.

Contents

Section Two
EXTRAS

Section Three
OPTIONS

Chapter 1

INTRODUCTION:
THE GOOD NEWS ABOUT SEX

You're holding in your hands the book I wish I had owned when I turned eighteen. I needed this book desperately, and believe me, things were much less complicated back then. I enjoyed the particular good fortunes of a unique place and time. Because I was brought up in an unconventional group-living situation by Buddhist parents in the Bay Area, my natural sexuality may not have gotten much direct encouragement at home, but my search for an authentic identity did. That, after all, was what had led my parents to Zen in the first place. Graduating from Berkeley High School in 1977, I came of age during the last decade when sexuality was widely considered a positive, healing, beautiful thing. The exposure I had to new ways of thinking about sex, "happiness," gender relations, culture, women's liberation, living arrangements, and personal responsibility supported my developing ideas about sex, men, women, and intimacy.

By the time I got naked with another for the first time, at the age of eighteen, I had read a good deal of the new thinking about social rules. Though from the beginning I was cautious and sensible in the way that parents would generally like their kids to be, my outlook on sex was broadly positive. I believed, and still believe, that my body is my friend and doesn't lie, that I must learn all I can about my physical self and take responsibility for my sexual satisfaction. When the time came, I felt safe to let my pleasure be my teacher.

Looking at the issues confronting young people today, I count myself blessed. They grew up with HIV-AIDS, abstinence-only "sex education," the bitter divisions of gender politics, and a social culture that sells them commodified sex in all forms while telling them not to engage in it. The heartfelt, confident, reassuring messages about sex that were common to my generation go all but unheard in theirs. For twenty years, the news about sex has all been bad.

But the good news, then and now, is that the truth about sex has never changed. Many, many people have managed to discover that truth, even in an era that hasn't made the search easy. That truth is there for you, and my message is that you are entitled to it. You are entitled to know your sexual self, express your sexual self, and satisfy your sexual self. You are also entitled to explore that self on your own or in the company of others. You are entitled not only to sex but also to thrilling, liberating, mind-blowing, soul-filling, intimacy-building total sex. You need never settle for less, and you shouldn't. The truth about sex is that it is yours by right. It is possible to become sexually sane, even in a culture torn with sexual insecurities. If I can do it, anyone can.

How do I know? Through twenty-five years as a sexual adventurer,

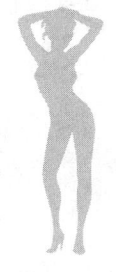

sex performer, sex activist, and sex educator, I've done the fieldwork and taken extensive notes. I've had "good" sex, "bad" sex, indifferent sex, funny sex, detached sex, angry sex, sad sex, clumsy sex, happy sex, romantic sex, wild sex, silly sex, transcendent sex, regrettable sex, seemed-like-a-good-idea-at-the-time sex, just about every kind of sex a person can have. I've had sex on camera well over a thousand times, with literally hundreds of different partners, all in addition to an active personal life brightened by a wide range of off-screen encounters.

In the adult entertainment business, I found a laboratory where I could conduct my experiments, a diverse pool of enthusiastic subjects, and a reliable subsidy for my research. With all pretenses of love and romance stripped away from the purely sexual interactions I sought out, I had the perfect situation in which to discover, as well as uncover, myself as a purely sexual being. For most, a situation requiring them to get naked and have sex with a stranger or strangers while other strangers took pictures would be, to put it mildly, profoundly intimidating. For me, such experiences were and still are exhilarating, deeply satisfying, and profoundly liberating. Professional, theatrical sex has been my classroom, a way into myself. Would I advocate this path for other seekers of sexual enlightenment? Probably not.

I'm often asked, "Why sex?" This is an imponderable of any purposeful life. Why art? Why medicine? Why mountain climbing? As my dad once put it, "Why not the violin?" There was no single character trait or person or incident that determined the direction I took, though there were certainly milestone moments. I just knew, by my late teens, that sexuality would always be my greatest fascination. This was well before I had dated, had sex, or even masturbated much. My instincts seem to have been correct. I'm very happy on my chosen path, despite its unavoidable bumps and detours.

Sex performance combines elements I've loved all my life: dance, movement, theater, feeling, emotion, plus lots of naked people. I had no idea how I'd make it into adult entertainment, but I knew the first time I saw an X-rated film in a movie theater that at least some of the answers I sought could be pursued in an environment of open sexual expression. Commercial pornography, which is all about hype and money, like any other branch of show business, didn't turn out to be the sexual utopia of my imagination, and I doubt that most sexually inquisitive individuals would find what they seek there. Once again, luck, timing, and a peculiarly well-adapted sensibility worked in my favor where others have been far less fortunate, and I feel it's important to express my gratitude by sharing what I've learned from my admittedly unorthodox form of amateur naturalism.

It's fair to say that my career in adult video has been a quest to answer these basic questions: Who am I sexually? What do I want? How do I talk about it? How do I make it real? What are the dangers and rewards of sexual activity? What do my desires say about me as a person? How can I feel at home in my body? Will I ever find a compatible mate? What the books I read didn't, and couldn't, do was address how to handle the complex, conflicted feelings that sex inevitably engenders. Starting from isolation and fear, how can we work through our beliefs surrounding sex and pleasure to arrive at love, community, compassion, and intimacy? After all my research, I have found a few answers.

I could pack a thick volume with colorful anecdotes from my career as a sex entertainer and yet another with my observations concerning pornography itself and its political, moral, and social implications in the wider world, but those books wouldn't help you. Just as I would had I pursued my likely alternative career choices as a nurse-midwife, I've found my greatest professional satisfaction in using my knowledge to

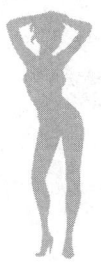

enable and empower others. Let's just say I've had all that sex so you won't necessarily have to.

It was my desire to share my understanding and insight with a world whose pain and confusion concerning sexuality I saw evidenced every day that gave rise to the instructional video series upon which this book is based. Adam&Eve, an adult-video production company with a sense of social mission similar to mine, approached me more than ten years ago to create an educational line with the purpose of providing explicitly detailed sexual instruction for adults. I started with the basics of oral sex, then went on to two very common interests, swinging and anal sex. The series is now in its thirtieth installment, having sold over half a million copies. I create each episode for "enthusiastic novices," individuals or couples wanting to improve their understanding and skill sets in the service of their own and their partners' sexual satisfaction. The phenomenal success of the video series testifies to the vast appetite for exactly this kind of specific, programmatic, supportive, informative approach to sexual learning.

Few readers will, themselves, attempt every practice described in this book, and the last thing I would want would be for anyone to feel pressured to try. I encourage you to take what you can, or want to, from my experience and use it to build your own erotic life, one that sustains and supports you on your terms.

Sexual Liberation: In and Out of Fashion but Always in Style

If there's one thing we've all found out during the past half century, it's that sex doesn't exist in a political vacuum. As a woman and a feminist, I developed my own sexual politics from the ideas of others and my own life experience. They're simple in theory but not always easily applied. They require rigorous honesty and a willingness to learn. I believe the body's innate capacity to experience sexual pleasure is an inherent good, requiring no validation by external authority, but I also understand that its power commands respect. My core position is that, between consenting adults, nothing short of physical harm is forbidden, no form of sexual activity inherently immoral. For that to be true, consent has to be real. Consent is not the absence of "no." It is a statement of shared intent and a contract that must be continually renewed. Every party to an act must fully understand and willfully choose to participate. Within those parameters, all choices should be honored. That's been my message for more than twenty years, and I'm sticking with it.

These beliefs have broad implications from which I don't shy away. I believe that all women must have complete access to the full spectrum of reproductive choice. Without control over fertility, women cannot be equal partners in sexual self-realization, as nature makes the stakes so much higher for us. I believe all consenting adults have the right to private pleasure without fear of governmental intrusion or hostile social scrutiny. As you would expect, I consider the viewing of erotic materials part of that sacrosanct zone of private pleasure. I do not believe that all sexual relationships are, or should be, struggles for political power. We all have a say in how political we allow the personal to become.

Sexual liberation requires that we take full responsibility for our actions and intentions and that no outside agency of church, state, or social organization should be allowed to do that for us. I believe that sexual jealousy is not "natural" but learned and that it can also be unlearned. I believe that we each have within us all the love and joy we

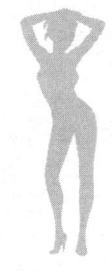

need (with plenty left over to share with others) and that only fear and conditioning prevent us from accessing these feelings. I believe that our bodies and our feelings, if honored and trusted, can lead us to our best lives, despite our diverse backgrounds. I realize that these ideas have been vigorously challenged from many quarters. Though I've submitted my own thinking to the test of daily life and the ongoing examination of what Zen calls "the beginner's mind," I remain an unabashed sexual liberationist in the broadest sense. My agenda is not hidden.

Sex, in its purely physical expression, has no intrinsic meaning. We, as adults, must give it meaning each and every time we choose to be intimate with one another. The beauty of the body is that it has its own wisdom, its own language, and its own timetable. Physiology has no "right" or "wrong." Friction on the flesh produces the release of neurotransmitters that, in turn, stimulate regions in the brain. Our skin is our largest organ. Not only does it keep our insides in and pathogens out, it also transmits sensations, and some square inches are more sensitive to attention than others. Caring touch keeps infants healthy, and lack of touch will create a condition known as "failure to thrive," a potentially life-threatening syndrome most commonly seen in institutionalized children, though it can occur in any child lacking adequate care.

Only through touch do we learn at the most basic, nonverbal level that we are loved, safe, and important to our caregivers. How we are touched in infancy and early childhood directly affects the development of our brains, particularly the ability to form healthy attachments in later life. It's not just essential in childhood; we need it all through life. In adulthood, one form that need takes is erotic desire. It's inevitable, eternal, purposeful, and precious. It's also anarchic, distracting, subversive, and frequently quite selfish.

Every culture has rules and limitations surrounding sexual behavior, though we often fail to take that into account when are own choices are in question. In our search for personally satisfying erotic lives, we must understand how the culture of our childhood affects us today. Was it particularly modest? Free and open about nudity? Judgmental of unconventional sexualities? Shame based? Fear based? Did it stress conformity or encourage individuality?

All through life, emotional connection starts with physical contact, though the dominant "romantic" conception of relationships as constructed by our culture insists otherwise. When we open up our exploration of sex, we find it infinitely more complex and nuanced than we ever imagined. Many forces are in play when we allow ourselves to be sexual, and we need to be aware of their influences. While sex itself may be "natural," in humans, all sexual behavior is learned.

In order to be whole, we can and must learn what kind of sexual expression is authentic for us and own it, choose for ourselves what restraints to put on it, and ultimately make peace with it. I believe that this happens anyway, whether consciously or not, which is why consciousness is so important. Human beings have proven miraculously resistant to ferocious external pressures on their sexuality. Western civilization has inveighed against the sinful excesses of sexuality for centuries and seen no reduction in them whatsoever. Clearly, like it or not, individual sexual choice will always be in individual hands, and that's exactly where I think it belongs. I put my faith in the basic good intentions and good sense of human beings when it comes to sex.

It's worth every tear, every struggle, and every heartache to make peace with our sexual selves, even if we never choose to share our bodies. When we are truly centered in this way, we no longer fear the opinions of others or need to judge what others do. Our first and most important relationship is with ourselves, and coming to terms with our bodies is

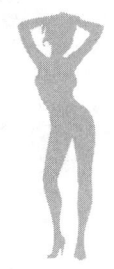

the cornerstone of that relationship. Grounded in self-acceptance, we can build healthy relationships based on love and respect instead of desperation and deceit. There is much more on the line than momentary pleasure. While total sex is a legitimate end in itself, its most important function is as a strong foundation for emotional intimacy. That is its ultimate satisfaction.

When I talk about total sex, I don't just mean totally hot sex or totally rockin' sex, though these are certainly desirable goals in themselves. I mean sex that involves us totally, encompassing all the biological and emotional forces at work inside that remarkably sensitive envelope through which we feel the physical world. That's the kind of sex I've learned to have, and you can, too.

Chapter 2

USING THIS BOOK

Looking at the list of chapter titles in the Contents, you'll probably see some topics that intrigue you, some that have the opposite effect, some that seem familiar, and some that seem to have originated in an alternative universe. How should you approach this daunting inventory of sexual possibilities? I suggest you do so in whatever way makes you most comfortable. What a few dedicated sexual pioneers may be tempted to regard as a blueprint is really intended as a road map. You choose the destinations, and the map shows you how to get there. You may find yourself taking in some unexpectedly interesting sights along the way, may elect to go the scenic route, or may head straight for the place you feel most at home. While a wide knowledge of the geography of sex enriches any life, you don't have to

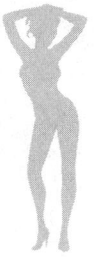

cover every millimeter of it in person. Obviously, not every topic covered in this book will resonate with every reader. As with sex in real life, you'll decide what's relevant to your life and what isn't.

Like any other journey, this one starts where you are. Before you find yourself in a room with anybody else, someone is already there. That's the person we need to know first before making contact with another. To find a compatible partner, you will need to understand your own sexual type. And I don't mean "stereotype" either. I'm not talking about an image you project or that others project onto you. I'm not even talking about who you think you are. I'm talking about who you really are, the critical elements of your sexual identity, which is itself a product of how and where you grew up, the beliefs and opinions to which you were exposed, the impact of your own experience, and some indeterminate component of your DNA that makes green your favorite color or accounts for your mysterious love of licorice. By the time you reach adulthood, you still may not know much about sex but will have formed desires and aversions nonetheless. Some will be as individual as a fingerprint; others will be the products of received wisdom, subject to modification with experience.

Your prospects for a fulfilling sex life have everything to do with your choice of a partner or partners, and how effectively you make that choice has everything to do with how well you understand your sexual self. Setting aside your aspirations for the moment, consider your influences, starting with the sexually chaotic culture you either grew up in or have joined.

If you associate words like *sin, hell,* and *damnation* with sex, you've got lots of company. And if the awareness of that language somehow adds to the thrill of your sexual adventures from time to time, you're not alone there, either. To the eternal frustration of lawmakers everywhere, attempts to inculcate restrictive sexual values aren't predictable, but we do feel their impact. We need to know which parts of our past conditioning we want to keep and which obstruct our search for intimacy and happiness.

For those who come to America as adults or whose parents are from another country, American attitudes toward sex are a migraine-inducing enigma. American sex culture is paradoxical in the extreme, characterized by a stubborn puritanical streak awkwardly wed to an equally robust embrace of personal freedom and casual hedonism. I can't tell you how to reconcile these contradictions. As a native, I continue to juggle them. No matter where we're from, it's incumbent on us, as adults, to invent our intimate lives, and though our freedom to do so here is always under attack, we're still fortunate to enjoy the personal liberties that our individualist character demands. Freedom is habit-forming, given time. Meanwhile, just don't tell your mother what you like to do on weekends!

We interpret our society's chaotic notions of sexuality through the lenses of our differing situations: where we grew up, our birth order, our educational opportunities, our aptitudes for making friends, and, most crucially, our interactions with adults. I was a somewhat shy, bespectacled, dreamy kid in braids and overalls who loved theater and drama but felt more comfortable working backstage in school plays. My parents had what I would describe as generally liberal attitudes about sex, but the subject was never discussed in any detail. I was enormously curious about sex and certainly put in the research hours at the library, but, contrary to what some might expect, the tolerant climate in which I grew up didn't precipitate my curiosity to early action. I was a fairly late starter and far from bold at the beginning.

But enough about me. It's your history that's important here.

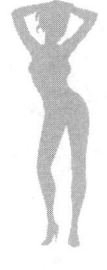

Where you're headed has a lot to do with where you started. Were your parents happily monogamous? Were they physically affectionate with each other? What expectations of a partner did your observations of them inspire? When and how did you first come to conceive of yourself as a sexual being? Granting that most early experimentations with sex are awkward, were yours exciting? Were they disappointing? Did they lead to unwanted consequences? Somehow, you got to the point of being willing to pick up this book. How did that happen?

Consider your present self. Are you in a monogamous relationship? Do you want to be? Are you looking to enhance an already satisfying sex life or to revitalize one that's lacking? How high a priority do you assign to sex in relation to your life's other concerns? Can you be casual about sex, or must it be in the context of a committed relationship? Are you inclined toward reserve and convention, or are you curious and venturesome? Are your appetites straightforward and easily satisfied or complex and demanding? In the absolute freedom of your fantasies, what are the elements to which you return for maximum excitement again and again? Is there a particular physical type to which you are inexorably drawn? Do you ever experience desire for your own gender or for multiple partners? How well do you know your own anatomy, and how comfortable are you with it? You'll need to answer these questions honestly, because the quiz is coming right up.

The practice you acquire by candidly addressing your own sexual identity will be vital to establishing an erotic link with a compatible other. Sooner or later, you will need to ask these questions of somebody else and be able to respect truthful responses, even when they aren't what you want to hear. If, for example, you know yourself to be monog-amously inclined, resolutely heterosexual, and wary of the unfamiliar, that fabulously charismatic, daring, omnisexual, polyamorous sexual dynamo you find so fascinating is probably wrong for you, and reading every page of this book isn't going to fix that. Likewise, if you're someone who wants sex every night, is turned on by the thought of watching your partner have an orgasm with somebody else, and feels strangely drawn to equestrian tack, your high school sweetheart who thinks of sex mainly in terms of making babies may not be your sexual type.

If not, nothing you or the object of your desire attempts will change this reality. You can both be fine people but not meant for each other. Clinging to an unsuitable partner in the forlorn hope that you will somehow adapt to each other when you're basically mismatched is a formula for permanent unhappiness. I stayed too long in an unhappy marriage because I was unwilling and unable to accept the fact that we were fundamentally sexually incompatible, and that nothing could alter that truth.

To have the sex that's right for you, you need to be the right person having sex with the right person. That's the most difficult sexual wisdom to attain and the part I can help you with the least. Most of that work is left to you.

Thankfully, the rest is teachable, learnable, and not rocket science. Once you've thought through what you really want to learn about and the purpose that learning will serve in your life, you can wander through these pages at will, checking out topics of incidental interest while pursuing in greater depth those that feel relevant to the sex life you want to have. I've done my best to lay out as broad a map as I can for you, and I don't expect you to cover it all at once or necessarily in its entirety.

That said, before you tick off the chapter titles that pique your interest, there are a few things you'll need to know for the trip, wherever you're ultimately headed.

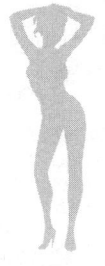

The Fundamental Things Apply

There are some truths that are always relevant when we're being sexual with another, whether it be our monogamous partner or a room full of naked people. It's no accident that I no longer ever have "bad" sex. No matter where, with whom, or under what circumstances I participate in sexual activity, I maintain rigorous discipline over my behaviors and choices, ensuring a reliably pleasurable time for all and no unintended consequences afterward. By scrupulous adherence to basic ethical standards, I can always look myself in the mirror after an erotic encounter, even if my partner's name escapes me. These precepts must be observed before the first kiss or the removal of the first article of clothing:

Safer Sex

1 *No laying on of hands,* much less any other body part, without full and complete agreement, the kind of real (as opposed to manipulated or engineered) consent we've already defined. There's no wiggle room in this matter. It's unethical and disrespectful to be anything less than candid regarding your expectations of a sexual encounter. Only full disclosure warrants the trust required for real sexual intimacy. If you want oral sex, learn how to ask for it. You may not push your partner's head into your lap and hope for the best. If you want to fuck your partner in the butt, you'll need to have that discussion before you slap on the lube. No getting the other person loaded to see "how far you can go." Men are more often accused of playing fast and loose with consent, but women are no less capable of doing so. Hanging all over your best friend's husband at the office Christmas party and then claiming later you were too wasted to know what you were doing won't work any better as an alibi for you than it will for him. And while we're on that subject . . .

2 *Don't be drunk or high.* Drugs and alcohol numb sensation, contribute to poor choices of partner or activity, and increase the odds of unsafe behavior. Most important, they remove the ability to give true consent. Lack of resistance from an inebriated person is, rightly, not a legal defense against charges of rape. And if you have to get baked to do something yourself, you just aren't ready for it, period. I'm not a purist when it comes to sex, and I don't think absolute sobriety is a must. A glass of wine or other mild intoxicant can be an enhancement to sex for those not confronting issues of addiction. But if you're high enough to worry about driving, you're in no condition to steer your own or another person's body through the rapids of sex.

3 *Realistically assess the risks.* There's been a lot of talk these past twenty years about "safe sex." This is an oxymoron. Sex can be made safer, but becoming physically intimate is never risk free. Discussions of safer sex in contemporary society usually concern methods of protection against sexually transmitted diseases, and in the age of HIV, that is always a consideration. Certainly, in isolated encounters or the early phases of new relationships, barrier protections against the exchange of potentially infectious bodily fluids, namely blood and semen, are a must. I believe this caution can be taken to needless extremes. I don't believe dental dams and condoms are indispensable for nonejaculatory oral sex, for example, as cases of disease transmission by those practices are rare.

However, when it comes to penetrative intercourse, condoms are the way to go until the health status of new sex partners is established by conclusive medical testing. Reliable, inexpensive screening is widely

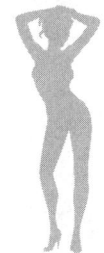

available, and if I were going to have sex with anyone more than once or twice, I would want to see my partner's test results and expect him or her to want the same from me. I realize a trip to the clinic together isn't exactly a romantic occasion, but it can create the opportunity for lots more worry-free hot dates in the future.

Here again, trust and honesty are vital if barrier protections are to be abandoned. Any STD test is only good for the day it was taken. If nonmonogamous partners then go out and have unprotected sex with strangers, they immediately invalidate the results. For highly active sexual seekers with multiple partners, regular and repeated testing is an ethical necessity, even if condoms or other barriers are used. While extremely effective against infection by HIV, syphilis, and gonorrhea, condoms aren't dependable defenses for chlamydia, HPV, and herpes. Ultimately, decisions concerning STD risk levels are among the most individual and personal we must make. There is no single regimen that works for everybody, and that is why I emphasize awareness as the key to maximizing safety. What you know must determine what you do. Nurse Nina says, "Get tested. Do it today."

Before moving on to happier subjects, we must also acknowledge that physical intimacy involves unknowns beyond the merely physical. Whenever we choose to open up to another, there is the chance that he or she may not reciprocate in kind. We may also be exposed to aspects of ourselves we're not prepared to face: our need, our loneliness, our desire, our fear, our judgments, and the unpredictability of our arousal. By being honest, both with our partners and ourselves, we can mitigate the dangers and amplify the benefits of sex, whether with only one partner or many.

4 *Listen to your instincts.* If you don't want to do a particular thing, don't do it. You need give no reason. You may not be able to put the feeling in the pit of your stomach into words, and you're not obligated. If your partner pushes or attempts to make you feel guilty, you should leave or at least get dressed. This is where the rubber of "self-respect" meets the road of "self-preservation." It doesn't matter if the other person gets mad at you; you need to care for yourself before anyone else can be expected to do so. Learning to recognize when your boundaries have been reached is the first step toward sexual autonomy.

5 *Learn all you can* about your unique sexuality and what does and does not satisfy it. Not knowing your own body's desires is certain to make an uncomfortable bed for you and anyone with whom you share it. You wouldn't buy an expensive sports car and then only let other people drive it. Make an operator's manual for your sexual self. Learn it on your own time. Masturbation isn't just a pleasant way to relieve stress; it's hands-on instruction. What you learn this way, you can pass on to others.

6 *Ask for what you want.* You can't read anybody else's mind, and nobody else can read yours, especially when you're sexually excited. This is especially important if you are new to each other. My husband and I don't have to talk much anymore, but we did, a lot, in the beginning of our relationship. I can't tell you how many hours I've wasted with others, lying in bed stiff as a board, wondering why somebody doesn't move to the left. How can he know to do so if I don't tell him? Learning to articulate my wants was one of the most important lessons of my own sex education.

7 *Be generous with both your partner and yourself.* You'll get as good as you give and vice versa. Sex isn't a competitive sport; don't withhold to make your partner "earn" your best efforts or go to the other extreme of trying to dazzle and outdo each other. Taking pleasure in our partners' pleasure is one of the joys and rewards of sex. Don't

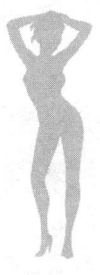

deny yourself that pleasure or deny it to others. If you don't feel the desire to please and be pleased with a particular person, you're in the wrong place, and it's time to go.

8 *Don't judge another's path to pleasure.* Deep and abiding intimacy occurs only in an atmosphere of acceptance and emotional safety. If what your lover wants isn't illegal (i.e., involving minors, family members, or livestock), try to have an open mind and heart. If it's definitely not on the menu for you, you're under no obligation to try it, even once, but strive to keep an open mind. You might be amazed at what you can learn to enjoy. When I realized that my judgments were a projection of my internal conflict, I was able to drop many of them.

9 *Take responsibility for your own feelings and the behaviors they provoke.* Sex play, whether between two people or twenty-two, is for grown-ups. Crying, dumping, whining, picking fights, or engaging in passive-aggressive manipulation has no place in the bedrooms of sexually aware adults. Sex triggers strong emotions, not all of them positive. Sex also makes us vulnerable to one another's expressions of those feelings. Know if you're refusing a request because it really isn't your thing or because you're throwing a silent tantrum and want to punish your partner. If you're having a true meltdown because something profoundly upsetting has been triggered, stop what you're doing and address the issue directly.

10 *Respect the process.* Sex is serious business, whether it's your wedding night or a casual playdate. If other people have set aside time in their schedules to be with you, be there. If you must cancel, give as much warning as you can, so they can do something else with their time. Demonstrate your appreciation of the importance of what you intend to share by showing up on time, looking and feeling your best, with a good attitude and good intentions. Sex should never be used to manipulate another or cause harm in any way, period. Spite fucks, mercy fucks, grudge fucks, and payback fucks are all bad fucks. Respect the power of sex and use it only for positive purposes.

This book covers a lot of territory, not all of which will be relevant to you. I suggest that you take the best (for you) and leave the rest. If you know yourself to be monogamous, don't worry about the chapters that include more than two people, though they may prove good fantasy fodder. If you run across a concept that intrigues you, but you feel you need to know more, consult the bibliography at the back of this book. If you have difficulty in speaking about something, you can point to a particular passage that addresses it to make discussion easier. If this book makes you sad, angry, or upset, be aware that strong emotions facilitate self-examination, which is always useful. All the decisions remain in your hands, whether or not you find the courage to take responsibility for them. The better informed those decisions, the greater your prospects for the outcomes you desire.

Now, let's get started. . . .

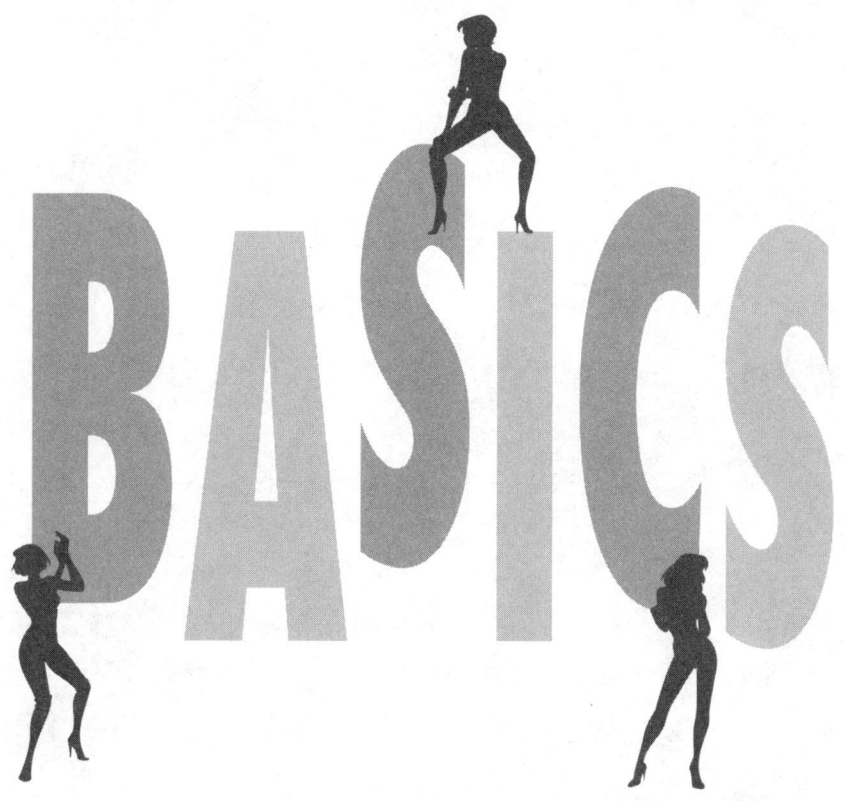

BASICS

Chapter 3

MASTURBATION:
FUN FOR ONE OR MORE

f Mother Nature hadn't wanted us to masturbate, she wouldn't have made our arms so long! Great sex starts with one person, and until that person learns to claim erotic pleasure for his or her own, sharing it with others is unlikely to realize its full potential. Sexual pleasure is an altered state of consciousness, resembling those produced by psychoactive drugs, through which we unleash powerful sensations of love, caring, intimacy, insight, security, and happiness. It's magical to be able to call up these feelings when we desire, independent of others, and then to apply what we learn to our enjoyment of sex with our partners.

As someone who has dedicated much of a career to inspiring masturbation—and undoubtedly creating some resentment from third parties for doing so—I remain convinced that an individual who hasn't learned to please him- or herself is unlikely to please anybody else. Masturbation is indispensable to sexual self-awareness, to basic understanding of physical pleasure, and quite possibly to sanity itself. And yet for all the masturbation I know to be in progress at this very moment, I'm well aware of the conflicted emotions that arise when we use our long arms for this utterly natural purpose. To get past those conflicted emotions, we need to understand how they arise.

Overcoming Negative Programming

Historically, religious and medical authorities (not to mention the Boy Scouts of America) have told us that "self-abuse" will buy us a one-way ticket to hell, sap our vitality, and grow hair on our palms. While our society may have advanced beyond the horrors of electrified antimasturbation belts and clitoridectomies once employed to deliver us from the menace of our simple desire to sexually self-soothe, more subtle sources of shame linger in our collective consciousness. Even many of us with no conscious negative judgment of masturbation per se are still inclined to view it as a poor substitute for "the real thing" or a somewhat pathetic analgesic to the pain of loneliness resulting from our inability to connect with appropriate partners. Common epithets like "jerk off" and "wanker" reveal the low esteem in which our culture holds those who find themselves "relegated" to this perfectly benign and quintessentially human activity. I'm happily married and lead a life of swashbuckling sexual adventure, but I still masturbate and don't intend to give it up anytime soon. I hardly think this indicates some deficit in my sex life.

I have my own suspicions regarding official and social hostility

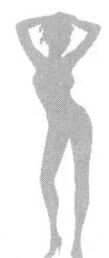

toward masturbation, which has everything to do with the political construction of sex as a subversive force that must be constrained for the maintenance of order and the preservation of existing power relationships. Frankly, a society that feels threatened by a bit of a wank now and then does not inspire my confidence. Such a society needs to get over itself, and so do we.

Whatever the sources of our shame about masturbation—rigid, authoritarian upbringings or unfortunate early experiences—we will have to overcome that shame if we are to understand and accept ourselves as sexual beings. Masturbation is self-love, not self-abuse, and until we accept it as such, we will lack understanding of the sexual activities needed to satisfy our own desires or those of others.

Masturbation is the first lovemaking skill you'll need to acquire, as it is the foundation of all others. While you may be born with the urge to do it, you aren't born knowing how. To become proficient at masturbation, you must familiarize yourself with your anatomy and its responses. Touch your genitals as often as you can. You're a grown-up now, and as long as you do so in private, there's no one to tell you not to. Be considerate of time and place, naturally, but do it: a moment here, two minutes there, every little bit helps. Pay attention to what feels good, and do more of it. Tastes in self-stimulation vary widely, and you'll discover your own by experimentation.

Creating Your Owner's Manual

The fantastic truth is that male and female genitals, for all their visible differences, are actually built on the same chassis. Until testosterone starts its work in fetal development to create a boy, all embryos are female, so it's no accident that our parts line up so well. If you're in possession of a factory-issue penis, you'll always have a clue as to what to do with a woman. The same goes for having a clitoris. The skin of a woman's outer labia is essentially similar to the tissue that makes up the scrotum. The skin of a woman's inner lips lines the male urethra. The clitoral hood is analogous to the foreskin on a man. Both the penis and clitoris are comprised of a shaft and a glans of erectile tissue. For men, the *frenum* (where the bottom of the glans connects with the shaft) and, for women, the *vestibule* (the super-smooth space between the clit and the vaginal opening or, in medical terms, the *introitus*) are the most sexually sensitive spots on the whole body. Both men and women are surprised to discover that the volume of erectile tissue in male and female genitals is roughly analogous: Women have just as much going on inside as men have going on outside.

Women have other sex/reproductive organs that don't correspond with men's in the same way (except for our gonads). Unlike the vagina, the uterus and fallopian tubes don't come into play during sex. The vagina is a strong, active, muscular organ equipped with lots of nerve bundles that respond favorably to penetration. The convergence of the inner labia close to the anus, the *fourchette,* is also highly sensitive to stimulation. But as a man's sexual pleasure begins with his penis, a woman's sexual pleasure originates in her clitoris, which responds simultaneously to direct stimulation and referred sensations from inside the vagina, home of the sometimes-elusive G-spot.

The G-spot, aka the *urethral sponge,* cushions the urinary tract during intercourse and also provides a "back door" to the clit. The clitoris turns out to be more extensive than just the shaft, glans, and hood visible outside of the body, with "legs" of erectile tissue embedded deep within the muscles surrounding the vaginal vault. Under adequate stimulation, the entire clitoris and surrounding pelvic muscles engorge

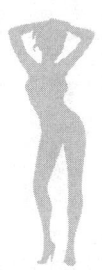

with blood, giving a woman an internal erection much akin to a man's external one. This internal erection, combined with secretions from vaginal glands, makes an aroused pussy plump, juicy, slick, springy, hungry, and ready for action.

Just as penises are offered in a wide range of sizes, so are vaginas, and, though they are famously accommodating, there is always an upper limit to the size of penis any one vagina finds enjoyable.

On men, between the scrotum and anus lies the bulb of the penis, where the penis is firmly and deeply attached, making an erection surprisingly sturdy. This is an excellent spot for squeezing, nuzzling, pressing, or rubbing, as it translates sensation to the super-sensitive *prostate gland* (also nicknamed the "P-spot") located behind the anal wall. This is a major source of erotic pleasure for many men. It can also be approached directly through anal play, which I'll address separately in a later chapter. Anal masturbation is common in both men and women and, with proper precautions regarding cleanliness and safety, can be an important enhancement to your repertoire of self-pleasing techniques.

As you explore your own geography in detail, you'll discover interesting individual anatomical quirks that you can learn to exploit to your own advantage, but the basic terrain is thoroughly mapped, waiting for your inquisitive touch to become well traveled.

Learning Your Own Process

Okay, so you've decided to become comfortable in your skin. Now what? Start with the body you have. Don't wait until you have the body you think you need in order to feel "sexy." As writer Mart Crowley famously observed, one great thing about masturbation is that you don't have to look your best. Each body is wired to feel pleasure right out of the box, including yours. Once you get to know and appreciate it, you can better assess how to display it to appeal to others.

The specifics of masturbation are relatively simple and primarily intuitive; you'll learn by doing. The sooner you start and the more frequently you practice, the more accomplished you'll become. While this advice could be taken to unhealthy extremes, in the form of compulsive masturbation that masks emotional problems, that concern is a remote one for most of us. The only consequence of masturbating "too much" is superficial irritation, which is likely to discourage overindulgence in the future. Men tend to masturbate more than women, understandably, given the impossibility of ignoring the evidence of masculine arousal, but I like to think women are catching up, and I encourage them to do so at every opportunity.

Still, it's important to realize that individual appetites vary enormously, and what seems like plenty of activity to some will feel like starvation to others. Our susceptibility to arousal isn't consistent either, rising and falling with circumstances, our emotional responses to them, and the cycles of our bodies. For example, while women's hormonal ups and downs may be more obvious than men's, both sexes' libidos fluctuate with the mix of chemicals in their bloodstreams. You'll determine for yourself how and how frequently masturbation fits into your daily routine.

Orgasmic response—the eventual though not inevitable purpose of most masturbation—is a spinal cord reflex. Think of it as a wired explosive charge with several detonators set to different timings. Each array of genital nerve endings needs a different type of stimulation of different duration to produce the explosive effect you desire. Some of us have "long pulls" before our orgasms can be triggered. For others, a few strokes

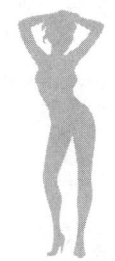

and it's "fire in the hole!" There are practical limits to how much you can control your body's basic response patterns, but one of the advantages of masturbation is the opportunity to explore those patterns in an unpressured environment. Eventual satisfaction is pretty much a given, so why not try a few variations once you've established favorite moves?

Precisely because masturbation is the one form of sexual behavior in which you can indulge with complete selfishness, you needn't ever feel that you should or shouldn't do so, as long as no horses are frightened. Of course, the more you enjoy the experience, the more frequently you're apt to desire it, and that is where the learned skill set of self-touch comes into play.

The Right Tools

You come pre-equipped with the most versatile tools for self-pleasing: your hands. When you touch your vulva or penis, you make the skin-on-skin contact for which everything else is a substitute. In familiarizing yourself with the operation of your own anatomy, you acquire a confident and instinctual understanding of the power of the intimate caress. I will return again and again to the critical importance of confident touch in the creation of the total sexual experience. That confident touch is first learned on our own bodies.

You'll soon discover that genitals are very sturdy things. While dangerous excesses have been attempted in the service of masturbation that might qualify as Darwin-award contenders, there is little risk of damage to your gear from regular, firm handling. While most of us are tentative with our own anatomies at first, eventually we're likely to appreciate a firm grip and/or a powerful friction as our comfort with our own sensations increases. Neither men nor women are particularly fragile (though they are highly sensitive) in their nether regions, which are engineered for hard use. If and when you reach the stage of masturbating with a partner, you will probably be surprised at how much more aggressively he or she handles the goods than you would when they're placed in your charge.

Fortunately, when it comes to the actual procedures, a single set of instructions works surprisingly well for both genders. A clit is essentially a miniature cock, something that women perceive as fully three-dimensional whose different regions respond to different stimulations. A penis is not merely a blunt object with little nuance but actually a giant clit that perceives infinite subtleties of touch. It's simply a matter of scale: millimeters versus inches. My husband, for whom worrying is a form of recreation, worries that this piece of volatile information will send both men and women into homophobic spins, but I have more confidence in you all. Knowing that men and women are more alike than different really should come as a relief to both.

If you women can pinch the bridge of your nose, you can grab your clit. For men, the equivalent would be to grab the whole shaft. For both, the sensation is reassuring and inspiring, a deep bass note on which to begin a symphony of sensations. Whether you place a fingertip at the base of your clit, pull your vulva up toward your navel and jerk it rhythmically, or seize your erection and stroke it at the ceiling, you'll experience a similar rush of blood to the region, accompanied by a stiffening of the erectile tissues. When a woman uses the heel of her hand to push her clit "into" her pussy, she feels the same sensation felt by a man when he pushes his hard-on toward his feet.

Stay with me here. When a woman places her thumb between her outer labia and thigh while keeping her fingers palm out on the other

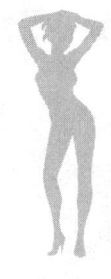

side of her vulva and "twangs" her lips and clit, she feels what a man feels when he strums his erection overhand, which partially explains why so many women in porn date bass players. They figure that if he can make this motion on a guitar, he can probably make it on her. Cupping the vulva with a thumb over the pubic bone and fingers at the *fourchette*, then squeezing while pulling the flesh away from the bone, produces a similar sensation to a man's stretching his package. Grabbing and pulling on the vulva with the heel of the hand rocking over the clit generates sensations similar to those created by milking the head of a cock from behind the corona.

Whatever the motion, start slowly and firmly, then allow yourself to be guided by the response. As you approach orgasm, you may need to speed up, slow down, or stop altogether to induce and prolong that perfect moment. Some people, most of them women, can come more than once during masturbation or lovemaking. Two to four orgasms are not uncommon, and I even know some lucky women who lose count after a while. If a man learns to separate ejaculation from orgasm (since they are separate physiological phenomena), he, too, can become multiorgasmic. As for myself, after many years of dedicated practice, I'm still stuck at one. It's gotten longer, stronger, and deeper, certainly, but rarely have I had more than one per session. I'm over it now, but I did feel inadequate for years. Later on, we'll take up the loaded topic of multiple orgasms, but when it comes to masturbatory enjoyment, there is no goal to seek beyond personal satisfaction. It's not a competitive sport.

However, masturbation is good exercise that strengthens the body for other sexual activities. The stronger your pelvic floor muscles become, the more powerful and controlled your orgasms will be. Try squeezing and releasing the muscles you would when attempting to hold back urination. Alternate squeezing hard for a ten-count with bursts of rapid squeezing and releasing. Do this in traffic, on the phone, and/or while listening to your boss drone on, and you'll be happy with the results.

While nothing surpasses the personal touch when it comes to masturbation, human ingenuity has never stood still in its attempts to improve on Nature. Dildos carved of wood, stone, or ivory turn up in archeological digs of sites from many different eras and places. The advent of modern technology has advanced the state of sex-toy art to impressive heights, of which you are the beneficiary.

The communal toy box now includes things that buzz (vibrators big and small), things that go inside (dildos and butt plugs, vibrating and non-), things that you can go inside of (jack-off sleeves, the molded vulvas of your favorite porn star), and things that wrap around strategic parts (ball stretchers, cock rings, and sheaths). Experimentation is required to find the items you like best, and it can get expensive, as toys are not returnable or exchangeable. Cheap toys are usually a big disappointment and will end up costing you more in the long run than an investment in good-quality tools for pleasure. I have a large collection of toys that don't work for me, and I still add to it from time to time. The desire for variety is understandable, but I return to my favorites over and over. In a subsequent chapter specifically devoted to sex toys, I'll get into some detail, but a few broad precepts seem to apply to masturbatory instruments in general.

In my experience, vibrating toys are less effective for men than women might expect, and penetrative toys are less effective for women than men might expect. For all our operational similarities, when it comes to interfacing with sex tech, the differences are fairly pronounced. Many women, myself among them, find a good, plug-in massager as indispensable to our great sex as a man's favorite brand of

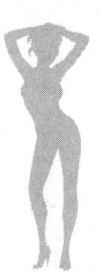

condom or lube is to his. Likewise, the kind of erotic imagery we use to excite our imaginations can diverge quite dramatically. It's common for both men and women to feel threatened or put off by each other's tastes in masturbatory aids. Why, we wonder, can't our partners (or even we ourselves) be satisfied with "the real thing"? I have no profound insight into Nature's plan, or even much confidence that such a plan exists, but my empirical observations suggest that men and women are just different enough in the operation of their orgasmic processes to require an element of active participation from both to achieve optimal results. One crucial lesson masturbation teaches us is that we can't hope for full satisfaction through complete passivity.

In addition to artificial sources of physical stimulation, the large and rather mysterious erogenous zone located between the ears is subject to arousal by viewing, reading, or listening to erotica in all its dizzying variety. Some of what's out there on the market, ranging from romance novels to the hardest gonzo video, will inspire your fantasies and ambitions. Much of what you see or hear will have exactly the opposite effect. Some prefer visual material, while others respond more enthusiastically to hot writing. Most people like to fantasize things that could, at least conceivably, happen in the real world. Others like to picture sex in completely fantastical settings involving practices only possible in the imagination. The important thing here is to discover the kind of sexual material that elicits your hottest response.

In your fantasies, you should enjoy complete freedom. There are no wrong thoughts, only wrong actions. Don't worry if what you imagine would be illegal or impossible if you actually tried to act it out; you won't be required to do so. Just as total sex requires the greatest respect for physical intimacy, it also requires that same respect for mental privacy. We may choose to share our fantasies with one another with total candor or to keep some inner thrills secret. This is not an issue of trust or loyalty. We demonstrate those qualities best when we are most accepting of our individual sexual identities, with all their quirks and contradictions. I think about all kinds of different things when I masturbate, and I assume my partners do, too. How much of that information we choose to share is the most personal of decisions.

Sharing the Experience

We tend to think of masturbation as a solitary, sometimes lonely pursuit, but it can also be a great addition to any couple's list of erotic options. Simultaneous masturbation is an all-fun/no-danger way to share enjoyment and get to know each other's preferences. As adults, we're free to engage in all the "heavy petting" of high school with none of the guilt and fear we felt at the time. For a newly dating couple, shared masturbation is sexy, daring, and safe, and it solves the irksome problems of what to do when you forgot to bring along a condom or you're still waiting for your test results from the clinic.

For established couples, sex is invariably enhanced when you're comfortable touching your own parts as well as each other's. Both men and women begin their masturbatory adventures in private, and many continue to feel self-conscious about how they will look to an observer in the throes of self-induced ecstasy. It's been my experience that both men and women find watching each other masturbate extremely stimulating and enjoy such a show far more than either might expect.

Many women and a significant number of men can't orgasm at all without rubbing their clits during intercourse or without giving themselves a few final strokes to trigger ejaculation. Remember that you have

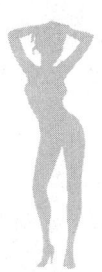

your own "operator's manual" for your individual processes of arousal and that it can only be beneficial to share the contents of that manual with each other. Rather than regarding the vibrator or the hand as "competition" during sex, try to accept each other's masturbatory participation as a cooperative effort that brings you closer together.

When intercourse isn't an option, masturbation can preserve the emotional contact between lovers. If you aren't "in the mood" and your significant other is, you can still assist, even if only with a bit of visual or verbal encouragement. This helps prevent naturally fluctuating sex drives from pushing you apart.

Ultimately, shared masturbation can and must build trust. When you expose yourself to another, you must know that your sharing is welcome, that you won't be ridiculed, and that, as they say about Las Vegas, what happens in the bedroom stays in the bedroom. Masturbation isn't a substitute for "the real thing"; it *is* the real thing. It involves real pleasure, real feelings, and real people.

Everyone has his or her own masturbatory style. It's very revealing to watch our partners masturbate. It gives us clues as to the kinds of stimulation they prefer. Does he like short strokes or long strokes? Does she rub her clit clockwise or counterclockwise? Does he like his balls held gently while he works his cock, or does he find the contact distracting? Does he enjoy pulling or stretching his scrotum? Does she like her breasts fondled as she fingers her pussy? All these little secrets bring us closer to our partners and help us to facilitate each other's enjoyment of sex.

Like any sexual pursuit, masturbation deserves to be treated with respect. Set up the bedroom as for any hot date, even if you're playing solo. Make sure you have all the things you'll need as the process unfolds. A full-length mirror situated so that you can easily see yourself (or -selves) can be a good prop. A bit of sexy costuming helps create an atmosphere of erotic potential, as opposed to utilitarian compromise. Start with kissing, petting, hugging, and grinding at a pace that feels relaxed and sexy. You can experience some of the thrill I feel as a performer for a special audience of one.

If, on the other hand, side-by-side or mutual action feels too much like a staged duet, take turns. You can show him or her how you like to be touched. Either of you can use a toy on the other, per his or her instructions. My husband often holds me while I work a vibrator on my clit. I feel close to him, and he doesn't have to manage all the minutia of my complicated orgasmic process, which helps me relax. Likewise, I can enjoy presenting whatever view of me he finds most enticing, providing my tits or ass to receive the tribute of his self-induced ejaculation.

Through masturbation you can discover much about your own sexuality and that of your partner, opening new avenues of shared pleasure when you overcome your shyness and learn to talk about how you please yourself. There is great reassurance in knowing that you can always satisfy or be satisfied. Secure in the awareness that you are always a great lover to yourself, you can't help feeling more confident as the lover of another.

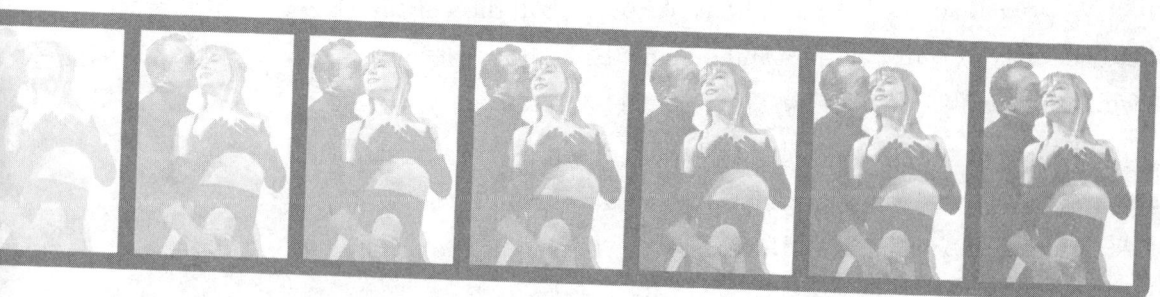

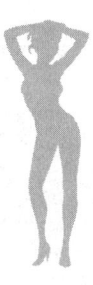

MASTURBATION MUST-HAVES

1 • *Privacy is a must.* 'Nuff said. Even if the goal is to become comfortable masturbating with a partner and seeing your partner masturbate, privacy is essential at first. You'll need to feel no pressure to "perform" a certain way or on a certain timetable, and you'll be able to recognize where you get in your own way.

2 • *There is no such thing as too much lube.* Nature won't always provide it for women, and women won't necessarily be able to provide it for men. I recommend flavorless, colorless, unscented lube for all sex, solo or otherwise. There are four basic formulations: water based, lotion style, silicone based, and petroleum based. Each is best for certain things. Water-based lube is easy on the body, condom compatible, and particularly excellent for women who are highly sensitive or who prefer to use silicone toys. The downside to water-based lube is that, with a lot of friction, it can become sticky. Refresh it with a few drops of water rather than adding more. Experiment with brands until you find the one that you like best. Lotion-style lubes are also usually water based but a bit thicker and not colorless. Some women love them, but I find they absorb more quickly than I like. Silicone-based lubes never get sticky and aren't absorbed by the skin. They're also expensive, but a little goes a long way. However, some people are allergic to them, so be alert for signs of irritation. Silicone lube is deadly to silicone toys. Always use condoms for that combo. Petroleum-based lubes are mainly used by men to masturbate, as they NEVER dry up or get sticky. However, they can't be used with condoms, as the oil will degrade the latex and you'll end up with a shredded rubber.

3 • *Use the right tools.* Once you find that perfect toy, you'll want it handy more often than not. Make sure you have it standing by, plugged in or charged up as needed; going off to search for an extension cord at the crucial moment is likely to put you out of the mood and will certainly have that effect on company.

4 • *Take basic precautions.* Gloves are a must for any butt play, as they prevent cross-contamination or nicks to the delicate tissue in the anus and rectum. They're also excellent for penetrative vaginal play, especially for women with long nails or men with rough skin.

5 • *Choose the appetizers.* You can use porn to remind yourself of things you already find exciting or to check out things that are new and different. In partnered masturbation, it's also useful to be able to point to an activity or device and say "That looks sexy," as opposed to actually having to make the suggestion. Try to be open-minded about the porn your partner likes. Shaming someone for what turns him or her on kills trust and intimacy. As I felt more at ease with my own sexual nature, I became comfortable with a wider range of pornography. Some things I used to like, I no longer do, and vice versa.

6 • *Create the atmosphere.* Thoughtful use of music, lighting, mirrors, candles, and the like all help us get over our initial discomfort over something that is both ordinary and extraordinary. Convenient placement of any gear you want is helpful. Turning off the phone and pager will ensure that you won't be interrupted at the wrong moment. Short of a bleeding child or fire, there's nothing going on in your life that can't wait thirty minutes.

7 • *Adjust your attitude.* If you already masturbate, use your time to develop your technique and learn to "surf" your pleasure waves. It takes discipline not to come when you first want to, but the experience will be deeper and stronger the more time you give to it. Men can learn to extend their preorgasmic period and even to become multiorgasmic, if they so desire. Women can learn to have longer, stronger orgasms. If you're new to this, you'll have to invest some energy in retraining and refocusing your mind. Your body is the guide in this endeavor, so follow its impulses, even if your chatty ego tries to sabotage your efforts.

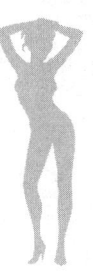

MASTURBATION MUST-NOTS

1 • *Lose all distractions.* You don't need the TV (unless you're watching your favorite XXX vid), the answering machine, or the voice from the computer telling you that you've got mail while you're trying to get your groove on. And you don't need unexpected visitors, so make sure your calendar is clear before you start.

2 • *No unwanted company.* If you're going solo, wait until spouses, kids, and other family members are out of the house. This experience is just for you. If you're masturbating with a partner, send the in-laws to a movie for the afternoon. And don't forget to put out the dog and/or cat; their help isn't required.

3 • *Avoid uncomfortable circumstances.* Whatever your hang-ups, they won't be assuaged by trying to masturbate while standing up in the hall closet or hunkering down in the backseat of your car in the garage. You need someplace safe and relaxing to explore self-pleasing.

4 • *Set no time limits.* How long should you allow yourself to get off? As long as it takes. Don't disrespect your own satisfaction by scheduling important tasks too close to your playtime.

5 • *Hang up your hang-ups.* Overcoming the shame and anxiety that's been conditioned into all of us regarding our need to comfort and satisfy ourselves isn't easy. You'll need to park all the negative lessons you've been taught at the bedroom door if you're going to enjoy your masturbatory experience.

6 • *Make no judgments.* Before you share self-stimulation with a partner, make certain that the ground rules are understood and that there will be no hostility or disapproval expressed, regardless of how you or your playmate seeks particular forms of release.

7 • *Forget goals.* Your only measure of success is enjoyment. Masturbatory pleasure isn't about how many orgasms you can have, how long they take, what you need to do to achieve them, or how they compare to what you've seen in pictures. Do what you like for as long as you like, moving on when you please and stopping when you've had enough. There is no standard you must live up to.

Chapter 4

THE GLORY OF O

Looked at from a distance, orgasm is as odd and alien a concept as anything science fiction could devise. Orgasm, as we know it, once euphemistically described in medical literature as "hysterical paroxysm," is unique to our species. It's not strictly necessary for reproductive purposes. It's not predictable, not always easily achieved, and not necessarily amenable to the same processes for both genders. It's fraught with emotion, and the having, or not, of orgasms is a frequent topic of discord between lovers. And yet, so ecstatic and satisfying is the orgasm that we pursue it with ferocious dedication and often at considerable risk and/or cost. Clearly, orgasm represents a lot more than the few moments of neurophysiological release by which it's clinically defined. While ultimately among the most authentically visceral sensations we experience in life, orgasm both gratifies and confounds us in ways that transcend our biology.

While only male ejaculation is required for procreation, women have developed a complex biology and anatomy that enable orgasmic capabilities of which many men are envious. I don't think for a moment that evolution would have invested such resources in selecting for these intricate mechanisms if they weren't adaptations needed for our species' survival. Shared orgasms help cement the pair bond and make the difficult and challenging work of intimacy worthwhile. Though ultimately personal, individual, and selfish, orgasms also provide us with a means of showing both generosity and appreciation to our partners. Their incidental benefits promote restful sleep, improve cardiovascular health, and contribute immeasurably to our emotional well-being. Could we do without them? Though it's entirely possible to enjoy sex play without coming (I do so, myself, on many occasions), orgasms are nature's way of ensuring our continuing motivation as sexual beings. They are, for most people, the ultimate reward that keeps the cycle of desire and fulfillment fired up and ready for action.

What an Orgasm Is and What It Isn't

Orgasms aren't magic, though they certainly can be magical, and we can't "give" them to our partners. We can only help make it safe for our partners to discover them while we help in any way we can. Like sex in general, orgasms have no intrinsic meaning or morality but are part and parcel of our existence as human animals. Sexual pleasure and orgasm are altered states of consciousness, akin to the psychedelic experience. An EEG (electroencephalograph) machine cannot

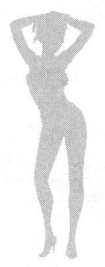

distinguish between brain activity during an ecstatic state induced sexually from one induced religiously. Like other bodily functions, such as digestion or blood-pressure regulation, orgasm is a function for which our bodies are wired, given the right situation and stimulation.

A sophisticated network of nerves connects our genitals to our brains, accounting for the depth and variety of sensations that good sex can elicit as well as the many different types of orgasms we can experience. The pudendal nerve is connected to both the penile and clitoral glans as well as the PC (pubococcygeus) muscle. The PC is a muscular "hammock" that holds our insides in, and having a strong one is very important to an individual's enjoyment of sex. The stronger the PC muscle, the better a person's control over his or her orgasm, and the exercises that strengthen it are named after the gynecologist who identified its usefulness: Kegels. The pelvic nerve lights up the clitoral shaft, clitoral legs, G-spot, bladder, uterus, and cervix in women while exciting responses in the penile shaft, testicles, and prostate gland in men. The hypogastric and vagus nerves receive input from the uterus, cervix, and anus in women and from the prostate and anus in men. That's a lot of specialized wiring that enables us to enjoy sex as no other creature in nature can in a comparable manner, in addition to which we have the unique capacity to enhance sexual pleasure consciously through the operation of our brain's cognitive processes. And, as is untrue among most other mammals, all these processes operate 24/7, three hundred sixty-five days a year. It's not surprising that anthropologists attribute the extraordinary success we humans have enjoyed in propagating ourselves on this planet to our unparalleled capacity for erotic satisfaction. The means by which we achieve orgasm may or may not seem "natural," but there can be little doubt that our ability to do so is.

Understanding the Cycle

Only during the past few decades has human sexual response been studied in a scientific manner, but we have learned a great deal about how the orgasmic process "works" in operational terms. It's generally agreed that our response cycle breaks down into four phases: excitement, plateau, orgasm, and resolution.

During the *excitement phase,* we become both physically and psychologically aroused: Nipples get hard, clitoral engorgement and vaginal lubrication begin to occur in women and penile erection in men, breathing quickens, and mental activity is stimulated. Other secondary effects, like flushed skin, perspiration, rapid heartbeat, and a sensation of increased body temperature, are also common.

Once we're aroused, the *plateau phase* can last from moments to an hour or more. As a general rule, it's easier for women to sustain an hour at the plateau than it is for men, though plenty of men have learned excellent self-control, and others have naturally "long-pull" triggers. While traversing the plateau, we masturbate or fuck toward rising levels of arousal and lowered inhibitions to release. As we'll discuss, with practice it's possible to maintain this enjoyable state for longer intervals.

Orgasm, climax, petit mort, *coming,* or whatever term you prefer represents the peak of the bell curve. This phase is characterized by muscle spasms; powerful, rhythmic, pulsating contractions of the uterus or prostate, urethra, and PC muscles lasting up to thirty seconds; generalized trembling; sensations of heat and cold; heavy breathing; spontaneous verbalizations; intense sensations of erotic pleasure centered in the genitalia but often felt throughout the body; and, in the vast majority of men and quite a few women, the expulsion of ejaculate through the urethra.

After orgasm itself comes the *resolution phase* (or the refractory

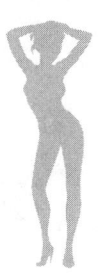

phase, as it's sometimes called), during which the body returns to its previous, unexcited state. For men, during resolution, another erection is impossible for anywhere from twenty minutes to twenty-four hours. Men's resolution phases generally become longer with age, unless the man has learned how to separate ejaculation from orgasm (more on that later). For women who are able to have more than one orgasm during a lovemaking session—women who are often described as "multiorgasmic"—the resolution phase can last mere moments, in some instances actually becoming shorter with each successive orgasm. I'm much like the average dude in that I rarely come more than once during a single lovemaking session, though I still consider my orgasmic response a work in progress.

Any number of factors can affect any part of the cycle. If you're distracted by anything from a ringing telephone to lingering doubts about your partner's affections, the excitement phase may take longer or fail to develop fully. If the physical stimulation applied isn't correct or the emotional connection is conflicted, the plateau phase may progress in fits and starts. If the orgasm is rushed or forced, its intensity and duration may be diminished. Under any of these conditions, the resolution phase, instead of being relaxed and comfy, might end up an emotional battleground or minefield. Though you can't control all these variables in every situation, what you bring to the process has a potent influence over how you experience the results.

The best component you can contribute to a shared orgasmic encounter is a thorough understanding of your own pleasure cycle. This is where masturbation is a most effective experimental method. What kinds of things excite you? Pictures? Stories? Poems? Music? Fantasies? Dancing? Necking? Petting? If you're alone, you'll have to imagine some of these things, but you'll eventually discover, in the well-stocked laboratory of your imagination, what elements enhance your response.

During the plateau phase, what kinds of stimulation do you like best? You can try rubbing and stroking; firm and light pressure; lotions, oils, and lubes; textures (fur, velvet, feathers, etc.); combining genital with anal or nipple stimulation; and vibrators and other sex toys, such as those we'll discuss a bit later. You can attempt to shorten or lengthen your plateaus by increasing or decreasing the intensity of self-stimulation.

With practice, you'll find subtle variations of orgasmic release: sharp, rolling, diffuse, localized, sparkly, explosive, or languid, to list just a few adjectives I've found myself using from time to time. As you're cresting over into orgasm, do you prefer the stimulation to speed up? Slow down? Lighten up? Get heavier? Go shallower or deeper? Strike a particular combination of stimulation and stick with it? Or do you prefer a combination of sensations?

During your resolution phase you may be very energetic or totally spent and sleepy. You may find yourself ready to go again right away, wanting more the more you get, or you may be ready for a nap. You may find yourself feeling particularly vulnerable emotionally. Orgasms release powerful pent-up emotions as well as *endorphins,* the body's natural intoxicants, thus lowering your threshold of inhibition to expressing withheld feelings. Tears, laughter, even anger are not uncommon manifestations of those feelings. Similarly, orgasm releases a flood of *oxytocin,* the chemical "bonding agent" that inspires powerful affections and the desire to attach, the natural chemistry that tends to make us feel like falling madly, passionately in love with someone after a good, strong climax, even though in a more rational state we might be inclined toward a more measured and sensible evaluation of our urge to attach to a particular partner. It's perfectly okay to fall in love with someone after such intense, shared enjoyment and perfectly reasonable to have second thoughts later in a moment of cool reflection.

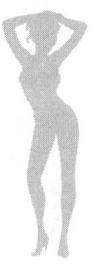

While any of these phases can be influenced by your partner and can change over time, with deliberate practice or by accident (as after surgery or becoming a parent), most of us eventually develop predictable patterns of orgasmic response that can only be altered, if at all, with great effort and distress. You may be able to come in a way that's different from what you're used to, and it can be fun to pursue that goal in a leisurely fashion, but there is no cause to see your particular cycle as somehow limiting or inadequate simply because it's predictable. You have a right to enjoy your orgasms to the fullest in the way that works best for you. Anybody who dares to denigrate your personal pleasure cycle doesn't deserve to be in your bed. And your own negative judgments regarding your particular preferences are more likely to obstruct your ability to expand your range of orgasmic options than to liberate them.

Just as your physical cycle is unique, so are your emotional needs during the phases of excitement and release. You may never want or need a close, emotional connection with a partner as you scale the orgasmic heights, even finding such intimacy distracting, or you may require a highly personal contact each and every time. Most of us are somewhere in between these poles, sharing the orgasmic experience with our partners to some extent, while inhabiting our own senses or playing our own internal film loops at the same time. Self-awareness is the paramount necessity in choosing a compatible partner, so pay attention to your emotional state when you come.

Taking the Pressure Off

While our individual physiological processes are what they are, it's often hard to sort out what's what, because of our prior conditioning concerning sex and our bodies. Sex is natural, yes, but no culture has what I'd call a "natural" sexuality, since dictating sexual conduct is a worldwide and millennia-old method of social control to enforce conformity. In the postindustrial West, sexual expression in general and orgasm in particular have taken on a political edge (in addition to their moral and/or religious overtones) that doesn't help us at all. Received notions of "good," "bad," "right," "wrong," "selfish," "immature," "mature," or "politically correct" orgasms do nothing constructive for an individual or a couple.

I can't count the times I've worried about having the "wrong" type of orgasm, induced the "wrong" way, stimulated by the "wrong" fantasies. Or that I wasn't having the "right" type of orgasm stemming from the "right" situation with the "right" person doing the "right" thing. While most of my insecurities were internal, a few partners have done their best to contribute to them. I know I'm not alone in this predicament, as evidenced by the shelf full of orgasmic polemics to be found in any bookstore. Here again, politics has no constructive contribution to make in the bedroom. You and your partner are the sole arbiters of correctness when it comes to this most personal of interactions.

I don't underestimate the difficulty of coming to terms with what gets you off and fully embracing whatever that is. Many voices must be stilled for you to pay heed to your own whispered longings. Guilt and judgment stand by all your life, ready to offer up a million reasons why you can't/shouldn't/dare not give yourself permission to follow your pleasure where it takes you. Just remember that your body can't lie. Your conditioned self exists only in your mind and isn't "real" in the sense of your physical self. Pleasure keeps body and emotion together. The key to increasing the "punch" of your orgasm is to use breathing to remain present while you expand, incrementally, the length of time you can experience pleasure before pulling back to a more comfortable

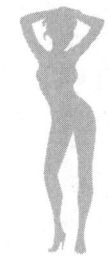

level. I began with being able to stay at my peak of pleasure for two seconds at most, and now I can last more than a minute. I taught myself to do it one second of claimed pleasure at a time, and you can, too. It takes patience and determination, but the insight gained through this exercise can be life-changing.

When you consider the varieties of orgasmic experience of which we might be capable, it's best not to measure them against one another according to whatever received notions have been inflicted by your upbringing, your education, or your previous partners. Try to think of orgasm in its many forms as a broad menu from which certain choices will suit your appetites better than others. As Oscar Wilde (who should certainly have known) once observed: In matters of taste, there can be no argument.

No Two Alike

Most men, and more women than porn would have us believe, usually experience one orgasm per lovemaking session. Their bodies don't need any more and/or can't go there again. I'm in this category. It takes me a long time to come, my orgasm is very intense and energetic (I look like I'm having some kind of seizure, I swear!), and I'm just exhausted by it afterward. On top of that, I find it uncomfortable and un-sexy to be touched after I come. My partners sometimes complain that I'm the one to fall asleep on them. A single orgasm may or may not be easy to achieve, but one is plenty satisfying to the person who has it. Whether from clitoral/penile stimulation alone or from a combination of internal and external sensations, the single orgasm is the norm, and you needn't feel less than fulfilled if that's all you want for a particular night.

In recent years, multiple orgasms, especially for women, have become a sort of goal unto themselves, a thing to be pursued by arduous labor if necessary and sorely missed if not attained. In fact, the capacity to come more than once in a given time period appears to be partially a learned response and partially an innate ability. Some women have resolution phases that last as little as five to twenty minutes, during which time they continue to enjoy intercourse or other sexual stimulation. They can climb completely up and down the four-phase orgasmic cycle two to five times in a session. Some need assistance from vibrators or other specialized forms of stimulation after the first one, or to get to the first one, and some don't. Some can do it just from fucking, and some need a combination of penetration and direct attention to the clitoris. Some women go easily back and forth between plateau and orgasm phases without descending into resolution and with each climax actually becoming easier until physical exhaustion finally sets in. Though I know from experience that such a partner can be quite an ego booster, I've learned that her response has more to do with her individual cycle than my abilities as a lover, which is one reason I don't feel pressured to attempt such feats myself.

Men who have mastered the technique of separating ejaculation from orgasm can also be multiorgasmic, though in a somewhat different way. They achieve peak sexual excitement, complete with the pulsating urethra and pelvic muscles (i.e., a "dry" orgasm), two to five times while making love, holding back on the "wet" finale until the end. It's quite a feat of discipline and dedication, and their partners are often quite appreciative, although, as with anything else, excess leads to irritation, literally in this instance. One of my playmates, who is in his fifties, has mastered this trick, and I must say he's a lot of fun, but I'm

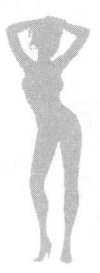

not sure how well I'd like a steady diet of such protracted penetration. Even men who don't actually learn how to be multiorgasmic can still benefit greatly from the exercises used in self-training, as they'll serve to extend the plateau phase to a mutually satisfying duration.

When a woman has an orgasm that combines both external and internal stimulation, thereby firing all of the nerves (pudendal, pelvic, hypogastric, and vagus) simultaneously, the result is a "blended" climax. While it's not often mentioned, a man can have a blended orgasm as well through prostate stimulation during intercourse, masturbation, or fellatio. These orgasms are usually very strong and satisfying. For many women, they are the only reliable kind. If you're one of those women, all talk of fusty, Freudian nonsense about "orgasmic immaturity" needs to be tossed out of the bedroom along with radical feminist cant about the essential "violation" of penetrative intercourse. Trust me, none of that stuff will help you get off.

A lot has been written in recent years about the G-spot, also called the urethral sponge or women's prostate. This pad of spongy tissue is located 1.5 to two inches inside the pussy along the top of the vaginal vault, where it surrounds and cushions the delicate urethra. With proper attention, the G-spot engorges and protrudes into the vaginal canal, where it can be felt easily. G-spots can be long, wide, narrow, short, firm, squishy, smooth, or bumpy. They're capable of secreting fluid into the urethra, which should come as no surprise since the G-spot's male anatomical equivalent, the prostate, also secretes fluid. Stimulating the G-spot with a finger, toy, or penis helps some women to come, while others complain that such ministrations merely produce urinary urgency. I think it's safe to say that for most women, some G-spot friction contributes greatly to the enjoyment of intercourse and accounts for the ability of many to orgasm from intercourse alone. I like penetration, including G-spot stimulation, but I can't climax from it alone.

While female ejaculation has become a trendy touchstone of feminine sexual liberation in recent years, it's not a new phenomenon by any means. Cultures around the world have celebrated these "feminine waters" since at least 600 B.C., mentioning it in texts both sacred and profane. However, it's only within the past thirty-five years or so, since the emergence of the most recent women's movement, that orgasm and sexual pleasure have been the subjects of open discussion, and female ejaculation has achieved somewhat symbolic status: the erotic equivalent of being able to write your name in the snow.

Some women have always squirted and not known what it was. Some have been mystified and mortified, as have their partners, at this messy spectacle, and other couples have always welcomed this evidence of a woman's enjoyment. As with men and multiple orgasms, many women can, if they want, learn how to squirt, with or without an accompanying orgasm, mainly by practiced autostimulation of the G-spot.

Physiology plays a role here, and women who can't externally ejaculate may be unable to do so because their urethral openings are set so deeply in their vaginas that any external expulsion of fluid is obstructed by the toy or penis. While there are some anatomical realities that make it less likely that a particular woman can learn how to squirt, a major impediment is psychological inhibition. To squirt, a woman must be able not just to masturbate, but to get messy, to let go, to risk what looks and feels much like peeing (even though the fluid expelled is procoital, not urinary) in the middle of sex, all of which are considered "unladylike." Female ejaculate is chemically different from

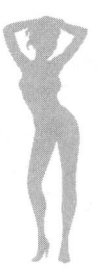

urine, so it's not a parlor trick. However, some of the more copious examples in porn videos are staged, so don't feel bad if you or your partner aren't as gushy and juicy as the ladies on your screen.

Unless a man has developed the ability to separate his orgasm from his ejaculation, he will automatically "squirt" when he comes, and this proof of orgasm is a focal point of most porn scenes. A lot of ink has been wasted telling us that most men get a macho or misogynist kick out of "marking" their territory in this way or that they see their messy orgasm as a way to humiliate or demean their female partners. I don't agree with this at all, individual jerks notwithstanding.

Ejaculation is a bodily function over which most men have very little control. It's just something their bodies do, and many are bewildered at the negative response their female partners have to it. To men, orgasms feel good, and they experience ejaculation as fun and pleasurable. Women who have been encouraged to see male sexuality as predatory, dirty, nasty, and without consciousness have an unjustified "ick" factor over a biological function. I don't like it when men get all skeeved out by the realities of menstruation, and I don't like it when women do the same over a few spurts of jizz. If you don't like ejaculate to get on your face or hair, let your man know to avoid those areas. It can be easily wiped up from anywhere else.

Male ejaculate is composed of fluid from several different glands: the testicles, the Cowper's glands, the seminal vesicles, and the prostate. Ejaculate can be clear, white, thin, thick, lumpy, goopy, or even chunky. These textural differences can be attributed to individual biology and the age of the man in question. A man can "shoot" or "dribble" his ejaculate, and this, too, is usually an individual biological variation among men. There is no correlation between the volume, texture, or force of a man's ejaculation and his state of arousal. I've been with guys who shoot five feet or more on a regular basis and men who dribble an inch. All enjoyed their orgasms immensely. If a man waits a few days between ejaculations, he'll have a bit more volume, and he may shoot farther, though it doesn't always work that way. Spermatozoa account for only about 10 percent of the total ejaculate, with the rest of the fluid comprising some thirty different compounds in trace amounts. The *seminal vesicles* produce most of the volume, and this fluid is rich in fructose, which nourishes the sperm until one of them finds an egg (or not). The fluid secreted by the prostate (about a third of the total volume) has an *alkaline pH,* which neutralizes the acidity of the vagina, so that the sperm don't die. This is why the ancient Roman methods of birth control—a bit of sea sponge soaked in vinegar or half a lemon placed in the vagina—weren't entirely ineffectual.

This alkaline pH is why semen tastes and/or smells like bleach and why it hurts like hell and makes your eye swell up if some gets into one. The *Cowper's glands* secrete a clear fluid called *preejaculate* or *precum,* which serves to clean out the urethra and to provide some additional lubrication. The longer a man spends getting turned on, the more of this he'll produce. It's equivalent to a woman's vaginal lubrication during arousal and can contain enough sperm to impregnate her, so be careful. The usual volume of ejaculate is approximately a teaspoon, give or take a few milliliters.

While male orgasms may appear to be a more straightforward proposition, literally, they vary in type and intensity as well, and men experience much of the same inner distress over them as women do. This is particularly true for men who are unable to prevent themselves from coming sooner than they wish, the dreaded premature ejaculation. Fortunately, a man can do a lot to lengthen his response time, using established physical techniques. It's true that some men certainly

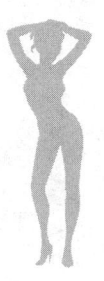

have short triggers, but many acquire masturbation habits when they're single that can get in the way when they're with a partner.

If you're jerking off only to relieve tension and get to sleep and you feel guilty about it to boot, you may develop the habit of rushing to the finish. I suggest you work at taking time to learn your process and extend your plateau phase, which will make you a more versatile lover. As you learn to identify the threshold twenty seconds before coming, you can alter the stimulation to avoid pulling the trigger. Try switching hands to change the stimulation or altering the rhythm of your stroke to distract yourself from impending orgasm.

With a partner, as you feel your orgasm building more quickly than you want, pull out and perform the tried-and-true "squeeze technique," grabbing or having your partner grab your cock behind the head and squeezing firmly for twenty to thirty seconds until the impulse passes. When you return to fucking, change it up a bit, altering the pace or changing positions. With a bit of practice, there should be no need to think about dead puppies or to recite batting averages backward in your head.

For some couples, simultaneous orgasm is the Holy Grail of climaxes, the moment when, literally, they "come together." Unfortunately, it's not much easier to find. Truly, this type of orgasm is extremely intense and pleasing, allowing both partners to boost their own energies with each other's. It's also very romantic and intimate. However, many people, myself included, have spent long, frustrating hours beating themselves up because they can't have this type of orgasm, or at least not consistently. If the two people involved have very different plateau phases or need very different types of stimulation, it can be nearly impossible to regularly achieve simultaneity, even if they love each other very much. I have had, during intercourse, exactly two—count 'em, two—simultaneous orgasms in the nearly thirty years I've been sexually active.

Keep in mind that good sex play is pleasure oriented, not goal oriented, so don't focus too much on it. Now, the most reliable simultaneous orgasms I have with my husband occur when I masturbate while he receives a blow job from one of our female playmates. No matter how you get to them, simultaneous orgasms are pretty great, but they're not the hallmark of successful lovemaking.

Finding Your Triggers

Whether simultaneous or not, orgasms during lovemaking are always cooperative ventures. I always ask a new partner what he or she needs from me when coming. One person's surefire get-off is another's ultimate annoyance. Some people like "dirty talk" all through sex, especially when going over the edge, whereas others need quiet to concentrate on sliding into home plate. One woman may get all dreamy and creamy when called a "slut," while another may abruptly stop and glare at you, breaking the magic mood. You can't tell by looking at a person what he or she likes, so ask!

And show yourself the same consideration by volunteering the little tricks that excite you the most: "I love it when my partner holds me down while I masturbate." "I love to be called a dirty boy/girl while I'm getting there." "Tell me how hot I am." You get the picture. As a rule, though, no one cares to be exhorted to come, as in "Oh yeah, come for me baby, yeah, that's it!" Talk about performance anxiety! If I have too much of you in my ear, my energy is not in my pussy, and we'll never get there. If you really must whisper the occasional encouragement, try sticking to a more neutral "Oh, you're so hot, that's so sexy," but keep it

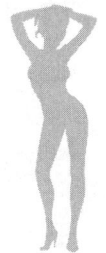

to a minimum. Sometimes, a partner may want you to say something with which you're not comfortable, especially if it involves a "bad" name, such as *slut* or *whore,* and you have the right to refuse. My view, not surprisingly, is that if it helps my partner to have more pleasure, what's the harm? I've grown a lot over the years by unloading some of my baggage at the behest of my lovers, and am happier for it.

The final few moments before orgasm can be dizzyingly ecstatic or freighted with anxiety and frustration. It's possible to reach the top of the orgasmic curve and still find yourself struggling for that last inch before the summit. This can happen to anybody for any number of reasons, virtually all of them psychological. The physical processes are well along by then, but your mind can still hold you back with inhibitions and insecurities of which you may not be aware until they kick in at this worst of all possible moments.

In order for the orgasmic cycle to complete itself, a final triggering mechanism has to kick in. Usually, it's a combination of physical sensation and mental activity. Just as your body is at its most fully present, your mind will often flash an image, a word, a few frames of your favorite fantasy that tip you over into climactic inevitability. Likewise, a momentary distraction; a sudden upwelling of guilt, anger, or shame; or an accidental wrong cue from a partner can make that tipping point maddeningly evasive. This is why it's so important to recognize your own orgasmic triggers and to be able to access them voluntarily. It is in the final countdown to blastoff that the importance of taking responsibility for your own orgasm becomes paramount. Whether this means communicating, verbally or otherwise, your need for something very specific to your partner or simply allowing yourself to go to that place in your head where you keep your most private "photo album," you still control the means by which you push yourself over the edge.

All of us come differently from different stimulation for different lengths of time, using different mental images to help us along. All of us must practice alone to get the best sense of ourselves, to come face-to-face with what it is that makes us hot. This is where we let our libidos lead us and disconnect our judging minds, the nagging ministers of our childhoods, scolding parents, or other shaming authority figures. Body and mind must work together with as little outside interference as possible.

A certain fantasy may push you over the edge every time, and it doesn't matter that it may be the same loop over and over. You have a mental slide show of fleeting images you flip through in your head. You may need a certain position to get that perfect edge: on hands and knees, kneeling over a vibrator or toy, or flat on your back. You may like to watch yourself in a mirror or need to have your eyes squeezed tightly shut. You may need a little assist from technology, as I do, or you may want your finale stripped to the simplest and most natural elements. There is no right or wrong way to come. Chances are there isn't much you can do to change the process by which the key synapses fire to ignite your climaxes or those of your partner.

Likewise, there is no cause to judge yourself or another by the specifics required. How long you take, what physical conditions you require, how hard you have to work for the desired results, and, above all, what goes on in your head at the time are all elements of your individual triggering mechanism and do not reflect who or what you are, sexually or otherwise. Some people fantasize about believable, attainable activities or partners, while others revel in extremes to which their imaginations can take them. Robert Louis Stevenson once remarked that every man has thoughts that would shock hell. As long as they re-

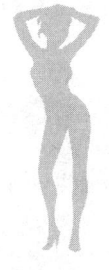

main mere thoughts, they are incapable of doing harm. I support full freedom of the imagination when it comes to getting off. Your brain needs no department of standards and practices telling it what to think as you invoke the shocking, politically incorrect vision that ignites your powder. You're not obligated to share the contents of your cortex with your other half, though it can be a wonderful, intimate form of emotional bonding to do so if you extend each other the acceptance that makes it safe to do so.

This is not to suggest that what your partner does in the final countdown to blastoff is irrelevant, particularly from a woman's point of view. Many women are what we call "preorgasmic," meaning that, well, they have not yet experienced orgasm, but it's the very rare man who has not had an orgasm by the time he's in high school. Barring a few seldom seen neurological conditions, a woman's preorgasmic state can reliably be attributed to social conditioning, since nearly all of us have the wiring necessary to come. It's a testament to the power of negative conditioning that so many women's minds are all that are keeping them from having the pleasure that is their birthright. These women certainly can benefit from private masturbatory explorations, but the right partner, along with a vibrator, can be extremely helpful—or not.

To overcome those internal barriers, a good partner must, above all, help create a space of protected intimacy in which no emotional pressures are applied and open communication is sincerely welcomed. If she wants to be talked through the experience, learn her language, or else be silent and supportive as she uses a vibrator, her hand, or your anatomy, as needed. Pay attention to changes in breathing and body posture that indicate increasing excitement and emphasize the activities that inspire those changes. Remember that penetration during orgasm is optional for many women, necessary for some, and counterproductive for others.

Take your lead from your partner. You're being of service during this stage, so your own ego needn't be involved. Just as she shouldn't beat herself up for not coming while you pump, it's no measure of your prowess if your dick is ultimately irrelevant to her climax. If she's brave enough to give you verbal cues ("harder, please," "to the left," "deeper," "slower," etc.), do your best to follow along. If you sense she's getting close, keep the rhythm that's working and don't speed up unless requested. Don't let your eagerness or arousal distract you from what she needs. As you get better at working together and communicating afterward about what helped and what didn't, you'll be able to do more with less talk and improve your ability to anticipate what's needed.

While the male orgasm is a somewhat more predictable phenomenon, it can still be enhanced or muted by a partner's behavior. Men also have preferences for preorgasmic stimulation that they may be shy of sharing. Some like harder, faster friction in the final strokes or a languid relaxation and heightened emotions. It may be difficult for a man to ask for his nipples to be pinched or for a finger in the anus at the last minute. As with women, some men like verbalizations, and others prefer quiet. His orgasm may not depend on these things, but it is in every way to both your advantage to be aware of them.

Despite any differences there may be between the genders when it comes to coming, I've found it to be true that in the final moments before orgasm (the proverbial "short strokes"), men and women prefer essentially the same treatment: They want the stimulation to continue just until they reach the peak of the orgasmic curve, when the contrac-

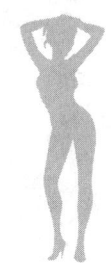

tions begin, followed by steady pressure until they stop. So, just squeeze the cock tightly, or press against the vulva firmly until the show is over (with men, tighten and relax your grip in time with the pulses. This "milks" him and feels great). Then rest your thigh on your partner's crotch until his or her breathing returns to normal. It's a lovely, sweet coda to a great ride.

After the Ball

In the warm afterglow of orgasm, we experience great satisfaction, relaxation, and a general opening of our senses. We also experience moments of extreme emotional vulnerability. In these unguarded moments, great romances can be born, and big mistakes can be made. We may have discovered the love of our lives, or we may simply be intoxicated with pleasure, increasing our susceptibility to impaired judgment.

Some men have complained to me that women "can't be casual about sex." I suspect that this is largely a matter of social conditioning, and my own observations suggest that it's becoming less true as women take control of their own sexuality, but it is a scientific fact that orgasm releases oxytocin, also called the "bonding hormone," in greater quantities in women than in men. It's also produced during childbirth, which helps a woman forget the pain and fall in love with her babies and may, in part, account for why women seem to fall in love with their partners seemingly more easily than do men.

Men, though a bit better defended hormonally, are far from immune to the potentially untoward aftereffects of an explosive climax. Men are capable of breathtaking self-delusion and denial when profoundly moved by what may be no more than a transitory physical experience. They have been known to exacerbate inappropriate bonding responses from women by suddenly uttering the "L" word when all they really meant to say was "Gee, that really felt great." They have also been observed to impute other qualities, ranging from profound wisdom to saintly virtue, to women of whom they know little more than a demonstrated ability to inspire a good pop.

Fortunately, both men and women are endowed with that higher brain function known as common sense, which can and should act as a break on the development of premature attachments to those with whom we may have no more in common than a particularly powerful sexual attraction and a shared ability to enjoy seismic orgasms. For all the joys that orgasms can produce, it's important for adults to recognize that, in and of themselves, they are the products of physical and mental processes, not magical miracles for which we must, or should, surrender our capacities for reasoned judgment.

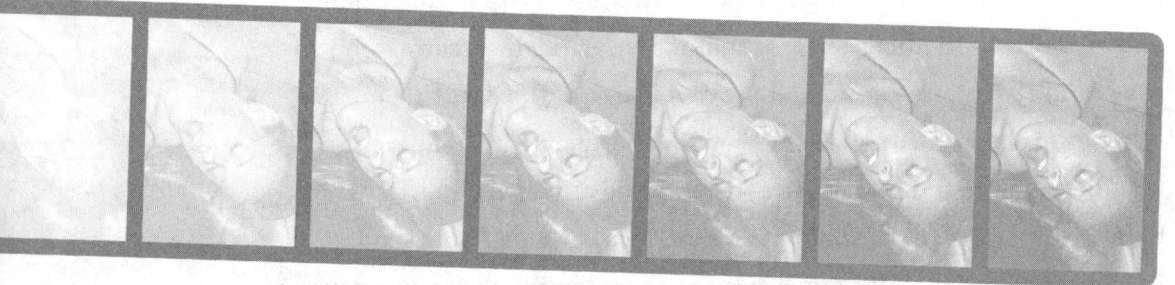

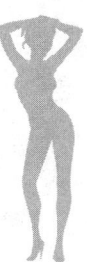

CLIMAX CLENCHERS

1 • *It's all about the journey.* Concentrate on enjoying the whole process, and the destination will take care of itself.

2 • *Own your pleasure.* Get to know what works for you and take responsibility for communicating this crucial information to your partner.

3 • *Create the space for pleasure.* Treat orgasmic pleasure with the respect it deserves by allowing time, space, and privacy to pursue it. Send the kids to the movies and turn off the phone.

4 • *Gather any tools you need.* It's no fun to fumble for a toy or a vibrator at the moment of truth. Make sure everything is within easy reach for you and/or your partner.

5 • *Do your homework.* Understand the physical mechanisms of orgasmic response, both your own and your partner's, and familiarize yourself with their operation.

6 • *Be adaptable.* If one thing isn't working, try something else.

7 • *Get involved.* Great orgasms take teamwork. If a bit of masturbation will help tip you over the edge, lend a hand.

8 • *Improvise.* You'll never know if a different position or fantasy scenario pumps up the orgasmic volume unless you try it.

SHOWSTOPPERS

1 • *No guilt trips.* You can't do much to change what gets you or your partner off, so accept yourself as you are and extend the same courtesy to your partner.

2 • *Forget keeping score.* Coming is not a competitive sport; it doesn't matter how many orgasms you have or how many you help induce. Quality is more important than quantity.

3 • *Don't push it.* You can't "make" somebody have an orgasm, but you can certainly annoy him or her by trying too hard. If it isn't happening at that moment, back off and wait for the mechanism to reset naturally.

4 • *Check your ego at the door.* If your partner doesn't respond with the screaming, furniture-breaking nut-buster you'd hoped for, don't take it personally. Everybody has moods.

5 • *Avoid excessive intoxication.* A glass of wine may lubricate the gears, but too much juice can cause the wheels to come off altogether.

6 • *Don't be afraid to ask for what you want.* Most people are relieved to know what works and what doesn't.

7 • *Never fake it.* A lover worth having won't be fooled but will be insulted.

8 • *Do not pretend to like what you don't or not to like what you do,* unless you want to spend a lifetime waiting for your partner to figure out the truth.

Chapter 5

FOREPLAY:
TURNING UP THE HEAT

Foreplay is everything—and I do mean everything—that leads up to sex. From the moment you and your partner decide to share a sexual encounter, all that you think, say, and do will contribute to the quality of that experience. In the broadest sense, a romantic dinner out, a candlelit half hour in the bath before you get started, a slow dance to your favorite music in the living room—all are foreplay. So are those little movies you run in your head about what's going to happen later. Before you've popped your first button, if you want your sex to live up to its full potential, you'll have kick-started the process in your own and each other's imaginations.

Let's assume, then, that the mood has been established and you've begun to sink into that lovely state of inevitability. You know for sure you're going to have sex, and you want to start out right. This is the moment when foreplay turns physical. From the first touch to the beginning of actual intercourse, there is a world of sensation to be mapped. The better you chart your course, the happier you'll be at your destination. Fortunately, the process is as pleasurable as the intended outcome, and that's how you should approach it. That's why it's called fore*play* as opposed to fore*work*. One less-than-positive aspect of the cookbook approach to sex instruction to which we've all been exposed over the past three decades has been the creation of a new syndrome I would call "foreplay insecurity": You've been told that everybody needs foreplay, that women in particular don't get enough of it, and that it's a list of must-dos to be followed like the Royal Canadian Air Force exercise program. It doesn't help that you see almost no physical foreplay in contemporary porn, yet in cable-TV soft-core erotica you see nothing else (and a highly stylized version at that). In short, foreplay has become political when it should be purely recreational.

So let's just take a deep breath here at the bedroom door and consider what you have to look forward to rather than what you think you're supposed to do next. First, you get to take an unhurried look at your partner with directly sexual intent, to really see the face and body of someone with whom you're about to be intimate. Now it's no longer impolite to admire a woman's cleavage or look hungrily at the bulge in a man's trousers; that's why you're here. From there, the process of discovery will become more direct. You'll be kissing, touching, undressing and helping your partner undress, exploring each other's anatomy visually and tactilely, experimenting with the sensations you can produce in each other, and learning to interpret the responses they provoke. As you approach the event horizon, your attention will focus more closely on genital stimulation until eventually you will be munching, sucking,

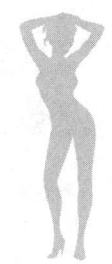

and fucking without any noticeable shifting of gears. Foreplay can take a long time, with much teasing and holding out to prolong the enjoyment of the preliminaries, or it can be compressed into a few moments of intense groping and fondling leading up to an abrupt, fast, and furious quickie. There are many routes to the same destination, and the secret of effective foreplay is choosing the correct one for the kind of ride you have in mind.

It's All "The Good Part"

While there certainly are exceptions, there seems to be a general division along gender lines over the concept of foreplay. Women want more warm-up, and men want to "get to the good part, already." While I usually think too much is made of gender differences and try to avoid taking sides where those differences appear, on this one, I'm with the ladies. As far as I'm concerned, once the process of sexual pleasure seeking begins, everything that follows is "the good part." Total sex requires an appreciation for the entire experience from start to finish. It does no good to resent what your partner needs to get in the mood to rip off your clothes. Those extra few minutes of focused attention are an investment in your own later satisfaction. Really, guys, what are you planning for the rest of your evening instead, ESPN?

Once you put aside the notion that sex equals intercourse, a whole new world of fun and pleasure opens up for all involved. The "good part" begins as soon as the lovers decide to share some fun. The only "goal" is mutual enjoyment, and that occurs all along the way to intercourse and even when fucking isn't an option. Dirty stories inspire much more fun when both parties are naked and one is sitting in the other's lap, their bodies in motion, acting out what's being read aloud. A woman loves to straddle a guy's thigh (why do you think men are called "hard legs"?) and squeeze away while acquainting herself with his cock and balls as he enjoys unobstructed access to her tits. Kissing and naughty talk are very effective here as well. Playing pool naked while "distracting" each other is a great way to work the voyeur-exhibitionist dynamic. Wrestling naked is a fantastic way to get adrenaline pumping as well as is flirting with hot pursuit-and-capture fantasies. Since men are usually bigger than women, though, negotiate how hard she likes to struggle or how "real" she prefers it to be, in order to avoid injury. Not feeling energetic enough for the WWF? Lie around reading the Sunday paper naked and see where it goes. This kind of foreplay is as much psychological as physical. It gives both parties permission to enjoy the pleasures to follow.

Secret of the Confident Touch

I have sex for a living. More often than not, I meet my coworkers for the first time only an hour or two before we do a scene together. Given that I might not have an emotional connection to my partners, there has to be a physical link or the scene won't fly. He won't get an erection, or she won't respond in a way that the camera can detect. I have less time to put this person at ease than "civilian" partners have to warm themselves and each other up, and (beyond a bit of flirtatious negotiation in the makeup room) only one means to do so: my touch. I put my practical familiarity with erotic physiology to use, and almost every one of my partners will report that, starting with the first laying on of hands, I'm a fun ride. While some people are born with this knack,

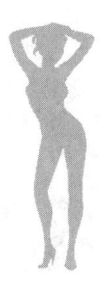

it can be acquired. You can learn to touch more effectively and inspire others to do likewise. You can't be a good lover without having good hands.

Much of what I needed to know about confident touching I first learned from my cat. Why a cat? Cats are beautiful, sensuous, and hedonistic, but what makes them so instructive is their utter lack of guilt. A cat won't tolerate any form of displeasure in order to be "polite," and that can be very revealing. When I was younger, I wondered why I had trouble keeping a cat in my lap. Eventually I understood that my uncertainty was transmitted to the animal through my hands. It could tell if I was tuned into its wavelength or not and responded accordingly. Slow, deep massage elicited relaxation while petting; respectful and attentive touching and scratching would make the cat go belly up and purr. This is where I learned to put aside my ego when it came to giving pleasure to others. The cat didn't care what I thought; it only knew what it felt. I had to learn to make my actions accurately reflect my intentions. That meant slowing down and letting go of goals and just enjoying the sensual pleasure of fur and purr on my lap.

When I first embrace a person, I slide my arm around his or her waist after a quick trip up his or her hip or butt before pulling him or her to me. My other hand can hold the back of the neck or drape across the shoulders or grasp a buttock or breast. Alternatively, that hand can reach down and cup the crotch of a lover. Pressing the heel of the hand into the base of a cock or clit feels fantastic to both parties, especially when combined with a firm but respectful package-grab. Hugging and grinding while your thighs are intertwined is an ageless method of arousing each other, especially while deep-kissing. When grabbing a butt cheek, slide your fingers to the place where the ass and leg meet, close in toward the anus, spread your fingers over a nice handful of flesh, and squeeze as you pull the cheek open. This teasingly stretches the anus in a delicious manner.

Human bodies are not fragile, and while a clumsy or rough touch can be downright repellent, a nervous or tentative touch sends a message of doubt and insecurity, which is equally off-putting. When you touch yourself during masturbation, you don't worry about whether you're doing it right or wrong; your body provides its own guidance. You do what comes naturally, and naturally you come. It is that same sense of easy familiarity that you want your touch to convey to your partner. What feels good to you probably feels good to him or her. Even if it's not ultimately the touch you'll perfect together, you'll have a good starting point from which to work.

Kissing Seals the Deal

Kissing is the spark that ignites my inner furnace, and without it I might as well masturbate. Regardless of physical appearance, I find a good kisser automatically more attractive and a bad kisser less so. The desire for oral satisfaction is as primal as desires get. Something warm and wet between our lips was the first sensual experience imprinted on our brains. Oral sensations are directly connected to the limbic system, the place in our brain that processes feeling and pleasure, love and satisfaction. Kissing brings us so close we can no longer see our partners and must rely on sensation.

How do you become a good kisser? First, find a good dentist and visit regularly. Practice proper oral hygiene. I shouldn't have to say this, but you'd be surprised at how many people are still fuzzy on the subject—literally. *Eww.*

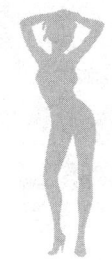

When I was younger and watching old movies on TV after school, I thought it was silly that the couple would kiss with closed mouths, often with their lips misaligned. Once I started kissing boys, though, I discovered that closed-mouth kissing generates a nice tingle without being intrusive. My appreciation for a bit of initial oral restraint increased as I began to encounter the kind of guy who tries to swab my throat as soon as he's within tongue reach. If I don't feel my partner tuning in to me, taking the time to seduce me, it's over. As with foreplay in general, don't rush the process.

To maintain spatial awareness when your eyes are closed, place one hand on your partner's cheek or at the junction of cheek and neck or at the back of the neck or head. With mouth closed, place your lips to your partner's, firmly but gently, letting the sensation wash over, and hold your partner's face to yours. Pressing harder, breathe in deeply, only releasing the pressure on his or her mouth and head at full inhalation, then pulling away a millimeter or two and exhaling. You will feel his or her body relax into yours, mouth softening, especially if you nuzzle his or her face for a breath or two. Repeat until a generalized sensation of languid familiarity replaces initial stiffness.

Usually, three or four applications will do it, but I continue for as long as I feel my partner's body pressing eagerly against mine. Each press-inhale/release-exhale cycle takes mere seconds, but these brief intervals set the tone of the lovemaking to follow. By his or her kisses, you'll know if your partner is fully present or in another time zone, wanting to pounce like a randy sailor or be seduced as a shy innocent. Take all the time you need here. Most sophisticated lovers I know, regardless of gender, can't get enough of good kissing. The more you kiss, the more you engender the desire to please.

When kissing a woman, it's polite to let her slip you some tongue first, allowing her to initiate instead of automatically making her the receptor. Do not try to perform a lingual tonsillectomy; nothing, and I do mean nothing, is more off-putting than battling what I call "cow tongue," that unpleasant sensation produced by a probing, slobbery, insensitive hunk o' snaky, mucilaginous muscle. Also, if your mouth happens to be a great deal bigger than your partner's, keep it closed enough to fit nicely with his or her lips to avoid that nasty drowning sensation.

Interspersing facial caressing and eye gazing with kissing increases the intimacy quotient. The key here is not to hide your true feelings. If you're scared, be scared. Your partner may be, too, or may be able to offer support. You're discovering each other as sexual beings, an awesome moment to which awe is a perfectly appropriate response. The closer in sync you are emotionally before you fuck, the better the experience will be, so take your time. The mood doesn't have to be overtly "romantic," but it does need to be authentic.

Hair, or sometimes the lack of it, is a sensitive matter with many people. My experience is that a person either loves to have it played with or loathes the prospect, so proceed with discretion as you approach the scalp of another. Once the green light is given, though, the proper combination of hair pulling and kissing can be positively swoon inducing. For enjoyable tugging, hair needs to be at least two inches long. Slide a flat, open hand up the back of the neck and into the hair, then simply make a fist and pull gently, allowing your partner's response to guide the intensity, speed, and duration of the traction. The back of the head and the crown make the best gripping points. Do not just reach out for some hair and grab it unless your idea of hot foreplay is a catfight. Combine hair pulling with kissing in this manner: The moment of hardest kiss and/or pull should be simultaneous, as should the release of both. If you're already squeezing or pressing the genitals, that pressure/release should sync up with the kissing and hair pulling as well. Try it and see for yourself!

Becoming Fluent in Body Language

As foreplay intensifies, your homework with masturbation becomes increasingly relevant. The confident touch you cultivated on yourself inspires confidence in others. One of my best lovers spoke not a word of English, and I knew no words of his native tongue. But just by touching and kissing, hugging and grinding, eye contact and smiling, we were able to share a fantastic few days and some of the best sex I've ever had, precisely because of the command we had of our respective bodies' intuitive responses, which was our lingua franca. Pleasure, the language of the body, is truly universal.

However, because the grammar you start with is your own, the syntax and vocabulary only yours, proceeding from monologue to dialogue often requires some translation beyond the purely physical. Before you get into bed with anyone, you'll need some discussion about boundaries, especially touch boundaries. Whether you intend to go the full distance to intercourse or to stop at any point along the way, you need to make clear what parts of your person are available for touching and in what manner. Be specific, neither apologetic nor antagonistic: "I want to be topless, and you can feel me through my jeans while I blow you," or "External anal play only; no penetration there until I know you better."

Likewise, you need to elicit this information from your partner. Don't accept "Oh, whatever you want is fine with me." Don't go forward until you both can state your limits and interests. Once these borders are drawn, they are not to be transgressed without either a direct invitation or further negotiation. If a sex partner can't be trusted to accept your limits regarding foreplay, you can be certain his or her manners will only deteriorate in more intimate circumstances. If a mild admonishment isn't sufficient to enforce the rules, it's time for somebody to get dressed and go home. One strike, and he or she is out. You'll thank and respect yourself in the morning (after giving yourself a big orgasm before bed).

I often start lovemaking with full-body hugging. It goes well with kissing, and the melting together of two bodies is a delicious moment. I have a way of hugging that brings good results with all my lovers. I embrace my partner and kiss as we find the best fit for our bodies. Then I squeeze firmly, smoothly ramping up the pressure until I've reached a point of maximum tension, followed by a quick release. I use the muscles of my upper back to pull him or her closer, and tighten my butt to provide a solid foundation and protect my lower back. It's a great workout! Rely on the response to guide how quickly, how hard, and how long to hold on. If he or she stiffens up, you've gone too far, too fast. If he or she hugs you back the same way, you're doing something right. If he or she melts and swoons, you're doing everything right. Don't be afraid to show your lover your strength! Done with care, it's almost always a big turn-on for your playmate. The combination of physical prowess and good manners is always a winning bet.

Pay close attention to breathing, yours and your partner's. Breathing together—literally conspiring—brings us close, so whenever I find myself not as connected with my partner as I'd like, kissing, hugging, and a touch of "conspiracy" will quickly get us back onto the same page, if not the same sentence. Between kisses, I like to take his or her head in my hand and turn it away from me. This exposes the ear and neck,

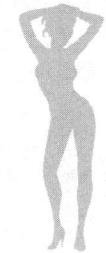

prime places of arousal and delight. Ears are very sensitive for most people, and touching them is usually relaxing. Avoid annoying ticklesome sensations and keep your tongue out of it, too. Pinch his or her earlobe firmly while pulling your fingers down it and twisting a bit. Suck on the lobe and drag your teeth over it. Go slowly enough so that each *ooh* and *ahh* registers. Without this distinct give-and-take, ear nibbling can be decidedly unsexy and irritating.

When biting the neck, location is everything. The best spot is on the shoulder close to where it meets the neck. Don't "nip" the skin. Use your parted teeth to press the muscles beneath, take a deep pinch of meat, squeeze your jaws quickly, pinch hard, and just as quickly release them as your partner exclaims, *"Ooh!"* in surprise. Combined with good hair pulling, this is a perennial favorite. If his or her nipples stiffen and you feel a slight shudder through both your bodies, you've scored a bull's-eye.

Chest fondling is also a nice way to turn up the heat. With a man, I'll pet, stroke, and squeeze his pectorals, touching his nipples as I ask him if they are erotically sensitive. If they are, I'll stay and amuse myself with them. The best way to fondle a woman's breast is firmly and confidently. Slide a hand up her rib cage until you cup the underside. Keeping the pressure firm, lift up her breast as far as it will go, until the skin is stretched tight over the glandular tissue within. With your thumb, rub and flick her nipple. This sensitive but confident approach lets her body know it's in capable hands. Squeezing both of her breasts together tightly feels good to both and creates the visual heaven known as cleavage, upon which you can gaze adoringly while speaking whatever truth moves you.

Depending on where a woman is in her cycle, breast or nipple play will either be the best thing since ice cream or the devil's own torment, so follow her lead. When it comes to nipples, success depends on fi-nesse. If you know how to roll spitballs, pull a piece of gum in two, nib-ble on a pencil eraser, or tune a radio dial, you know how to fondle nipples. When in doubt, have her suck and nibble on your earlobe the way she likes her nipples to be played with. The nerve distribution is very similar, and you'll totally get the idea. Women experience their nipples, like their clits, in three dimensions. Drag your teeth along the top, biting ever so subtly at the edge. With both hands, pinch the skin near the *areola* (the pigmented tissue around the nipple) and pull it up. Take her nipple between your teeth and slowly shake your head from side to side, scraping the wet nipple gently with the edge of your teeth pressed just tightly enough to make her moan. Twiddle the nipple while pulling on it, adding a little pinch here and there. As long as you know what you're doing, you can be surprisingly assertive. Just re-member to pay attention to the signals your partner sends back.

By the time I've reached the sitting-on-the-couch-and-kissing stage, I'm ready to add heavy petting to the mix. How you touch your part-ner's vital parts varies, depending on which hand you're using. For our discussion, the hand closest to your partner is the "near" one; the hand farthest away is the "off" one. With a man, I reach over using my off hand and place my thumb on the top of his cock, the tip touching his abdomen. If he's hard, I wrap my fingers underneath his cock, the back of my hand pressing firmly into the space between his cock and balls, and follow the ridge of his erection as far back as I can easily go. If he's not hard yet, my fingers naturally fit behind his scrotum, against the bulb of his penis. I alternate squeezing/pulling motions on his cock and scrotum with pressure/rubbing of the bulb. I use my thumb to pull his whole package back down toward his butt. His kissing usually gets more passionate as I alternate patterns, with him squeezing his pelvic

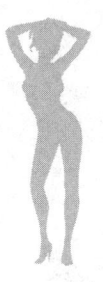

floor muscles in reply. The intensity of his response tells me when I'm on target.

Using my near hand, I can do the same thing by coming from above his cock instead of straight onto it. My thumb and fingers encircle his stuff, fondling and enjoying the meaty heft of him. From this angle, instead of pulling his cock down, I squeeze the bulb with my fingers and the top with my thumb and pull up and out in a milking rhythm: squeeze-lift/drop-press. If he's hard, I don't jerk his cock right away as much as pull it in different directions. Pulling the skin tight around his shaft and then shaking is the kind of move that would have guaranteed me plenty of dates in high school, had I known how to do it back then. Using the thumb and forefinger of my off hand, I pinch just the head of his cock until I feel the hard shaft right behind my grip as I pull on it.

By paying close attention to his body language during these experimental phases, I find my way to a working combination of squeezing and stroking that produces plenty of back arching and verbal encouragement. Once I find that formula, I stick with it. I may change up the speed or rhythm, but with either a male or female partner, it's important to establish that pleasantly stimulating touches will be repeated to achieve maximum arousal. Nothing is more frustrating than trying to relax into a hot groove and having your partner suddenly feel inspired to go for something completely different. Constant, repeated, dependable strokes build momentum for whatever is to follow. If you've explored partnered masturbation, you'll observe a pattern of hand moves that emerges as your partner becomes more aroused. The best thing you can do is emulate that pattern as closely as possible. When it comes to cocks, jerking is usually the basic stroke that gets the best results, whether as a work-up to intercourse or a preliminary to the Big Squirt. Personally, I get a lot of pleasure from diddling and twiddling with cocks, but I know that when it's time to get serious, firm and steady massaging pressure is the most consistently effective technique.

With a woman, I place my off hand at her pubic bone (where her clit starts) and firmly pinch her entire vulva between my thumb and fingers, moving them up and down her outer lips until I feel the unmistakable hardness of her clit and its glans. You'll know it when you find it, as she'll squeal/moan/melt/giggle/grind. You can't squeeze too hard here, as her lips provide all the protection and lubrication a clit could want. Pull her lips away from her pubic bone. With your thumb, push her clit through your first and second fingers and pull some more. Try to hold still, pinch steadily, and watch how she moves against your hand.

All too often, well-meaning men, eager to please, retract the tissue around the clit and stimulate it directly as if trying to erase it. Nerve endings are more concentrated in the head of the clit than over the length of the penis, so too much focus on too small a piece of real estate will produce more irritation than arousal. Working the clit through the labial tissue is a far more reliable turn-on. I've introduced this pinch-and-wiggle method to literally hundreds of men and women, and I've never had a complaint yet.

When using my near hand, I place my palm against a woman's pubic bone and pinch the entire vulva from above instead of from the front. The "spitball" method of vulvar manipulation, swirling her clit in delightful ways, is a surefire winner. You'll need to dig deep with your fingers, getting a good pinch, before bringing them together for squeezing and rolling, as if you're trying to reach behind the clit to pull it away from the body. Roll her clit under your thumb as if it were a small piece of wet paper. Each circle of the thumb is a full stroke for this tiny, concentrated bundle of receptors. Micromotion is the secret of pushing

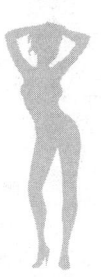

her buzz button with consistent success. The strokes may grow quite focused and intense as orgasm approaches, but the territory covered is likely to remain fairly small. Again, watching your female partner masturbate uninhibitedly is the best orientation you could hope for in making yourself welcome on this unfamiliar terrain.

With either gender, it's important to stay in touch with the whole body during foreplay rather than reducing it to a "parts shop." Keep an available hand on the neck of your partner, pull your mouth away from his or hers, and maintain eye contact while you rub those tender parts. Good foreplay is all about communication. All of us want to be seen when we're turned on and welcomed in that state, so now's the time to extend that acceptance. You're not a couple of mechanics stripping down an engine; you're collaborators in an experimental project.

When one has time to plan for an evening of pleasure, foreplay becomes even more fun and exciting. In addition to turning off phones and pagers, clear out all mundane, daily clutter, leaving behind only what you'll need: a sexy book or magazine, drinks, mood lighting, music, scented candles, etc. Set up the bed with what you know you'll need when you get there: toys, condoms, lube, gloves, baby wipes or a towel, mood lighting, music, etc. That way, the flow isn't interrupted or the mood broken by frantically searching at the last minute for something you missed. "Spontaneity" must be planned for.

While some couples really go all out in the sexy costume department and love role playing, most people are happy with some article of clothing that (1) makes them feel very sexy, and/or (2) is a tried-and-true turn-on for their partner. It may seem strange, but I've rarely met a man who doesn't just l-o-v-e a woman in a pair of black high heels and nothing else. I know it seems "porno," but there's a reason for it! Some men prefer pumps, some prefer mules, some like the addition of stockings, but almost all men like heels. Learning to walk in four- to five-inch heels is one of those sex skills that is well worth developing. There's nothing quite like high heels for enhancing the legs and making a woman feel, and be, super-feminine. Women are becoming more visual, so men should dress to provide pleasure as well. A man in a nice silk robe is always an eye-catcher for me! I like the casualness as well as the easy access to his naughty bits.

I'm comfortable with getting right down to heavy petting, but many people prefer to warm things up more slowly, and games are good for that. Your local adult novelty store will have lots to choose from: board games, card games, dice games, and combinations thereof. There are shelves of books devoted to sexy little games for lovers that you might want to check out for more ideas. Pick one that seems the most fun and playful, but ask your partner first. Chocolate-flavored body paint doesn't go well with someone who hates to get sticky and messy, and that's just one example of a potential mismatch.

I know that many people like to get a little "buzz" going as part of foreplay, using whatever intoxicant they prefer, and I have no philosophical problem with that, to a point. The rule of thumb here is that if you're too wasted to drive legally, you're too wasted to have good sex, especially with a new partner. Nothing is more of a letdown than my

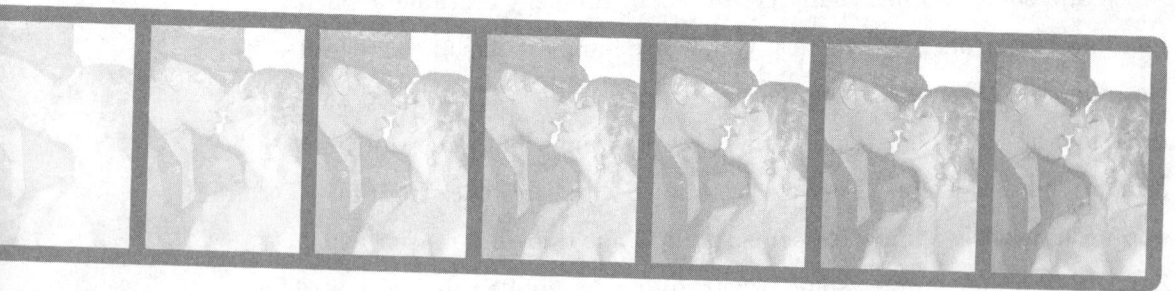

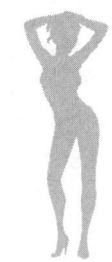

partner, out of nervousness or whatever, getting so drunk or high that he or she is no longer the person I was attracted to and wanted to play with. If you're nervous, be nervous. If you're scared, be scared. If you're having second thoughts, don't drown them out. Instead, heed them, even if it means stopping for the evening and going home. There is no honor in fucking an intoxicated person. It's no fun, and it might even be illegal.

Oral sex is such a big part of foreplay, I've devoted two whole chapters to it, so check out the one that's right for you.

FABULOUS FIRE STARTERS

1 • *Talk the talk.* Don't hesitate to tell your partner how attractive you find him or her. We're all insecure, and we all need encouragement.

2 • *Touch as you would be touched.* Don't be afraid to guide your partner's hands toward the places you want them and away from the places you don't.

3 • *Take your time.* A slow burn makes for a hot fire. Don't rush the process.

4 • *Make the first kiss a memorable one without forcing the issue;* you'll get only one.

5 • *Stick with what works.* When something you do produces a pleasurable sigh or shiver, do it again.

6 • *Allow yourself to enjoy being pleased.* There is as much skill in receiving as there is in giving.

7 • *Let your partner know what feels good.* You don't have to set off fireworks to signal your appreciation, but it never hurts to encourage more of the things you like.

8 • *Be helpful.* Two sets of hands are better than one. Most people enjoy watching their partners stimulate themselves.

9 • *Foreplay doesn't end when fucking begins.* Revisit pleasurable diversions throughout the process.

DEAL BREAKERS

1 • *Don't get to the point too soon.* You want to involve your partner's entire body. Going straight for the clit or dick defeats the purpose of foreplay.

2 • *Avoid falling into a routine.* The kiss-kiss-right-nipple/munch-munch-left-nipple approach leads to speculations about repainting the ceiling.

3 • *No keeping score.* Sometimes one person gets more attention than the other. Sometimes one person needs more attention than the other. Be cool with it.

4 • *Never pretend to like something you don't,* lest you end up with a whole lot more of it in the future.

5 • *Be careful not to ignore a subtle hint.* More obvious expressions of displeasure may follow.

6 • *Nobody likes a show-off.* Trying to impress a new lover with all your acquired skills is less effective than sincerely responding to his or her promptings.

7 • *Do not be stubborn about asking for directions.* You're not a mind reader; don't pretend you are.

8 • *No ripping of garments without prior consent.* Good lingerie isn't cheap.

Chapter 6

CUNNILINGUS:
WORKING UNDER THE HOOD

ne thing I can tell you as a happily bisexual woman is that if you're squeamish about pussy, it's likely to have the same response to you. Your willingness and ability to communicate your enthusiasm for feminine anatomy by way of oral stimulation may well be the most significant determinant of the degree of enthusiasm you inspire in those regions in return. It's impossible to be a good lover of women without being a skilled and ardent cunnilinguist. Whatever your excuses or hesitations when it comes to putting your face between a woman's legs, now's the time to get over them. If you think that a pussy is somehow "dirty," know that a freshly washed vulva is considerably cleaner than a human mouth, so if you're willing to kiss, you should have no problem with applying your lingual skills farther south. Insecurity about your technique is also a cop-out. No secret decoder ring is needed to decrypt the process of pleasing a woman through oral stimulation, only a willingness to learn some basic physiology and a few simple techniques. Rote routine, however, means little without the real desire to satisfy. If you resist pleasing your partner in this way, or do so grudgingly or ineptly, expect to see her taillights fade over the horizon after the second date.

Fortunately, there is no greater obstacle to mastering cunnilingus than your own hesitation, and the rewards for overcoming it are both immediate and long term. I've always been fascinated by pussies, starting with my own, and I've learned to make friends with all kinds of them. So can you, whatever the nature of your factory-issued equipment. Get ready to earn your diving certificate.

Inventory of Parts: They All Work

As happens with manual stimulation, the most common mistake of the eager novice is to focus too narrowly on what is assumed to be the most important piece of real estate. Every square millimeter of a woman's sexual anatomy is capable of responding to oral stimulation and will do so reliably if given half a chance. Going straight for the clit and licking, flicking, sucking, and slurping madly away at it is much more apt to produce irritation, both physical and emotional, than satisfaction. Let's start by reconnoitering the entire terrain, up close and personal.

There are five basic components of a woman's genitals that respond to oral stimulation: the labia, the clit, the vestibule, the *fourchette* (where her lips meet, near her anus) and surrounding musculature, and the vagina. Each requires something different to produce maximum arousal.

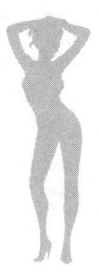

Lips like to be pinched between the teeth and pulled. They also like being sucked firmly. In addition to suction, clits take to being squeezed between the teeth. Be sure to keep the hood in place and gently scrape the shaft and glans with the edges of your teeth. Like the cut edge of an exposed cable, there are eight thousand exposed nerve endings in a clit, so the slooooow, gentle drag of a sharp, wet tooth edge is exquisitely intense. Covering your uppers with a hooked lip is never a bad idea. The vestibule, being the most sensitive part, needs gentle, moist contact. When taking a mouthful of pussy, your tongue will naturally rest there. Grasp the clit between your upper teeth and tongue and gently shake or nod your head, subtly stimulating the vestibule with each movement. The *fourchette* responds well to licking and the contact of your face pressed against it, stimulating the important muscles of the pelvic floor. Your tongue won't reach very far into the vagina, and it doesn't have to. As you press your face to the *fourchette*, your tongue will penetrate just far enough to stimulate the "itchy" nerves at the entrance. Wide, circular, lapping motions with a flat tongue feel good here too.

The crucial element to keep in mind is that all these parts operate in concert to produce an excited, and ultimately orgasmic, response. I often start with just my hands, massaging my partner's *fourchette* and the muscles around it until she's fully relaxed and starting to move her hips. Before seeking out all the hidden treasures, begin by taking the entire vulva into your mouth in a slow, powerful, sucking embrace with lips and tongue and working all that sensitive tissue around in leisurely swirls. You'll quickly discover—as with IKEA furniture—that no extra parts are included in the package; everything serves a purpose. Likewise, your own inventory includes more than one relevant subassembly. Mouths work best in concert with hands, and tongues can't do their best work without the support of knowing lips and teeth.

Only after I've massaged and petted all the parts I intend to stimulate do I put my mouth on a partner's clit, keeping the rhythms of mouth and hand in sync. I can apply suction with my mouth and let the massaging of the *fourchette* teasingly move her clit between my lips. When I put a thumb in her pussy and press downward, she relaxes her muscles, and when she contracts them, I let up on the pressure. If she's really bucking her hips, I don't try to "do" anything except maintain contact. I've found it most effective to start with one form of stimulation and get a groove going before adding the next one. Sensation builds slowly, layer upon layer, into a complex and satisfying whole. In our upcoming chapter "Making Love to Women," I'll delve into the specifics of hand-and-mouth coordination in greater detail.

If the intended mood is playful and teasing, spend time massaging and manipulating the labia, clitoral hood, and the muscles surrounding the vaginal opening until she's pulling at your hair or otherwise demonstrating her urgent need. Do things to her outer labia that men like having done to their scrotums: pulling, pinching, twisting, stretching, and tugging. Stretch her flesh slowly and firmly until she moans, breathes deeply, and relaxes visibly.

You must coax a woman into relaxing under your touch, since you can't ever "force" her to do so. If she's stiff or jerking away, you're not connecting and need to change your approach. Put an arm around her hip with your hand resting on her stomach, or reach up and grab a breast or her hand. The secret is to stick with any one move until you feel a response from her before making the next one. I use the rhythm of dancing to help me, since both foreplay and dancing are physical forms of communication that bypass the forebrain. If you can pay attention and do a basic four-count, you can perk up any pussy with a few minutes of focused attention.

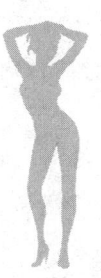

As the heat rises, I place my upper jaw across her pubic bone at the base of the clit and my lower jaw over the introitus (the vaginal opening). I rest the entire weight of my head on her mound and nuzzle slowly, applying the gentlest of suction, perhaps combined with the smallest of nodding motions. Breathing in, I pull the vulva into my mouth, releasing it as I exhale. I continue until I can tell she's breathing with me. It's easy to become riveted by the fascinating details of your closeup work, but you need to be aware of the whole body surrounding them. Breathing, pulse, verbal expressions, twitching and squirming, and the undulations of your partner's limbs are all indicators of the effects you're producing.

When her pussy is twitching very softly and regularly, I start to suck more intently, carefully pulling the clit away from the pubic bone as I pinch the flesh hard between my jaws, perhaps slowly "shaking" my head from side to side. All my movements are big and slow, so she can play along with them. The short version: Take a mouthful of pussy and gum it to death. The long version: Press the front teeth at the base of the clit, against the pubic bone, and suck it in firmly as you place the flat of the tongue against the vestibule, also firmly, and then don't move at all. Remember, clits are so sensitive that just her heartbeat and your breathing will stimulate hers fully.

Intersperse this with relentless, patient, methodical sucking of all of her pussy flesh for as long as she likes. Try little tricks with the tip of your tongue and see how she reacts. A high-pitched squeal tells me I'm coming on too strong, while a low growl suggests I'm doing something right. The less extra flesh you take into your mouth and the more you suck the clit itself, the more deliberate, wetter, slower, and tinier your movements have to be. Remember: With women, millimeters mean everything.

Something else that works well is to place your lower teeth at the base of the clit and, with your upper teeth, bite the flesh above her vulva as you move your chin toward her belly button an inch or two. This stretches her clit and feels fantastic. Don't bite too hard, and don't do this too quickly unless you want to hear a yelp and end up with a mouthful of wet sheet as your partner flees the bedroom. It will leave painless tooth marks, just so you know.

While porn has become a de facto form of sex instruction in a society that does a poor job of conveying technical specifics by other means, some of what it teaches is just plain wrong and needs to be unlearned by anyone wishing to please a fellow human, as opposed to emulating the formulaic acts of professional performers. Good cunnilingus is all but invisible to the observer, as it requires a tight seal of mouth on pussy and much more sucking than licking. The dreadful, open-mouthed, tongue flicking you see on video is meant to expose the action to the camera, not to be copied at home. The mark of good cunnilingual technique is an upper lip hooked down over the clit hood, with all the important action going on out of sight underneath.

Here's my simplest and best universal approach to cunnilingus under the widest variety of circumstances: When in doubt, apply pressure and leave it to her to supply the movement.

No Two Alike

Having learned to identify the universal anatomical landmarks, you can find your way around any pussy, even in the dark. Next up is learning to interpret the signs and signals our partners give us to guide our way and how to communicate in return. Each gasp, moan, hip thrust, grind, leg squeeze, and ear tug conveys useful intelligence.

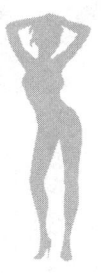

Far from being unknowable, pussies give clear signals, once we slow down enough to receive them.

While all women's bodies come with the same set of standard options, there is a vast diversity in the manner in which they operate. No amount of technical skill will guarantee you predictable results when you engage in the arts of oral pleasure. Every woman has unique physical characteristics and a range of individual emotional responses to go with them. Simply inflicting your best moves on your partner without paying close attention to how they're received is a shortcut to erotic annoyance. A pussy is part of a person, and how you relate to the rest of that person has as much to do with her enjoyment of your attentions as any physical thrills you might labor to induce.

Even though all pussies have the same parts, they vary greatly in appearance, which is part of their eternal charm for me. Some pussies form a wide V, and some a narrow one. Some mounds are fleshy, and some are bony. Some outer lips are fat and tight, with all the inner workings hidden behind a narrow cleft, while the inner lips of other vulvas spill out in abundance. Some clits are hardly visible, even with the lips pulled back, and some are an inch long, even when not aroused. Just as it's impossible to forecast the full volume of a man's erection by the size of his softie, it's impossible to tell how roomy a woman's vagina is by the appearance of her vulva.

With the increasing popularity of genital piercings, you may come across someone who has jewelry in delicate places. A piercing, especially of a woman's clit hood, may greatly enhance her ability to orgasm during penetration by giving her clit just the extra little tickle it needs, so it's not a bad thing. Your tongue will naturally play with the jewelry when you've sucked her clit into your mouth, so go with it. Bite it and pull, ever so slowly and gently, until she moans. Press the ring or barbell against her clit as you nod or shake your head, adding another dimension to the stimulation. If she has rings in either set of lips, use them to hold her pussy open like a valentine while you use your mouth on her.

Before you proceed to the sheer exhilaration and romance of wowing a woman with your oral skills, it's essential to keep in mind that each woman likes different stimulation at different times. Consistency in paying attention to her response is as critical to a positive outcome as what you do physically. What works perfectly for one woman may fall flat with another. What sends your partner through the ceiling at one moment (or time of the month) may send her to the freezer for ice cream a day later. In short, you can't use your mouth effectively unless it's properly wired to your brain and the rest of your senses.

Enthusiasm and Technique— You Get Points for Both

It took me years before I could easily remain in the moment with my partner during oral sex and fully appreciate the excitement of her pleasure. Unlike a penis, a hard clit and a relaxed one are almost the same size. There is an obvious, easily determined "standard" for effective fellatio. By contrast, even good cunnilingus may appear "boring," with "nothing much going on" at the point of contact. There is a natural tendency to lose focus in such ambiguous territory, and I'm as much subject to it as any other lover. When my concentration drifts, I refocus my attention on the pussy before me, again choosing to be my best, most centered, least neurotic self. Early on, I'd have to refocus a dozen times a minute. By learning to tune in to my partner's pleasure, I've trained my busy mind not to wander. The important cues are to be

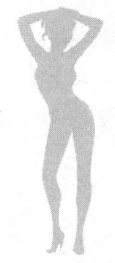

found in the woman's face and body, which show her reaction to what she's experiencing. I've been known to snake a hand up between her tits to feel for the pounding of a telltale heart and sweep my palm from side to side in search of erect nipples or the sheen from breaking sweat. I listen for changes in breathing and note the tensing of thigh muscles next to my face. These signals may not be as obvious as a throbbing chubby, but they add up to useful cues from which to take direction.

Cunnilingus is not something you do to your partner. It's something the two of you do together, and that's where we move beyond the realm of the purely mechanical. A woman's orgasmic response is both a reflexive, unique, hard-wired, physiological fact of life and a product of highly changeable emotional states. It knows no intrinsic right or wrong. Rather than take a woman's particular orgasmic requirements personally and reproach yourself or her for their unpredictability, learn from what you observe. Your desire to please is more important to the ultimate result than any tricks or treats you can pull out for the occasion.

With any one movement—sucking, swirling, biting, etc.—there are three aspects that are combined in an infinite number of combinations. These are the movement itself, the pressure one uses, and at what frequency (sixty times a minute, once every five seconds, etc.). So she may like what you're doing but wants you to change part of it—e.g., to keep sucking but to slow it down and do it harder, or to shake your head faster with a looser bite. You get the picture.

If there is a single secret to my pussy-eating talent, beyond my command of anatomy and physiology, it's the positive attitude I bring to it. By the time I'm on my stomach between a woman's legs, we're already pretty aroused and frisky. Having reached the limit of first gear with necking and petting, it's time to shift to second. I start by looking at her pussy and petting it as I describe the feelings it inspires: "It's beautiful." "It looks so juicy." "Wow, I'm nervous." "Your clit is so big already!" "Show me how you like to touch yourself." "Dirty talk" is just speaking the truth of the moment using the vernacular. It really helps to set the mood and bring the players closer together. However, a little goes a long way, so don't overdo it, lest you distract instead of inspire.

It doesn't matter how good I am at oral sex: If my partner doesn't communicate her desires, my powers lose their magic. A woman who actively participates in cunnilingus will get a lot more out of it than one who lies back passively, waiting for something to happen to her. Direct instructions such as "a little more to the left" or "ouch, too hard!" and the time-honored face-grinding/hair-and-ear-pulling method of signaling for more or less of whatever you're doing are helpful, but the most important means of communication are subtle and intimate. I tell my partner to squeeze her pussy whenever she'd like to yell, yelp, scream, beg, plead, or whimper. How and when she tightens and relaxes her pelvic muscles, rocks her hips, and arches her back speak directly to my mouth. How fast or how long I do any one thing depends on my lover's responses.

On the receiving end, where I'm equally happy and at ease, I experiment with different breathing/squeezing/relaxing/grinding combinations as my partner stimulates me orally. Redirecting the energy inward heightens the excitement and intensifies my experience, which is then expressed through the natural movements of my excited body. I've found that too much thrashing and screaming can be a way of hiding the fact that somebody's not really present or having a good time. I never pretend to enjoy something I don't; such deceptions ultimately show disrespect for good intentions and perpetuate bad habits.

If I need to be more in control, particularly with a willing but inexperienced partner, I sit astride his or her face. If my partner simply

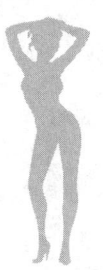

sucks in a lot of flesh, my own grinding and rocking will pull and tug on my clit until I find a groove that works for me. The best mouth position for this is the same one we make when we bite into a perfectly ripe peach, just before the juice starts to run down our chins.

As a woman who enjoys receiving oral sex, I keep my vulva neat and clean. Bare skin transmits sensation more effectively and subtly than fuzzy flesh, so shaving the outer lips is an easy way to enhance the pleasures of cunnilingus. I'm aware that the "hair-versus-bare" debate has passionate partisans on both sides and that personal fetishes and political convictions complicate the question. Certainly, this is a matter of individual discretion, and suggestions from lovers are best couched in the most diplomatic language possible.

However, I don't hold with the view that those who prefer more exposed terrain secretly harbor pedophilic urges or have been conditioned by porn to reject a woman's "natural" appearance. It is normal to groom oneself to make sexual relations more appealing. My politics in this regard are purely hedonistic. I can't physically tolerate the abrasion of a man's coarse facial stubble (and aesthetically dislike the "fashionably unshaven" look), so I unhesitatingly issue razors to male partners and send them off to the bathroom before allowing them to go down on me. I make it clear that it's not their faces I'm rejecting, merely their excess foliage, and I would take no offense at a similar suggestion from someone planning to explore my own nether regions. Once again, I would stress that the bedroom is not an ideal forum for sociopolitical analysis of body-image issues. Overall, it's been my experience that women who trim, shave, or style their pubic hair report a higher degree of body comfort than those who don't, but my sampling is profoundly unscientific.

At the same time, there's no reason to regard your own or another's genitals as inherently unsightly or unappetizing and therefore in need of compulsive grooming. Avoid the use of perfumes or douches, especially those with fragrance. A clean vulva is the most appealing (no one eats pussy to get a taste of Mountain Lilac). Perfume is bitter to the taste, and scented douches tend to irritate membranes and foster yeast infections.

The key point to keep in mind in regard to cunnilingus, as with any other form of sexual activity, is that both partners do everything they can to physically and psychologically facilitate comfort and intimacy and do nothing to elicit the opposite effect. The right attitude and the relevant anatomical parts in good working order create the atmosphere in which mutual satisfaction is most consistently achieved.

What's In It for You?

Having made it clear that I personally love to eat pussy and that overall I believe lovers should do what they enjoy and not feel pressured to do what they don't enjoy, what is to be said to those who simply don't find oral sex appealing for whatever reasons and would rather not engage in it? My answer isn't exactly PC, but that's never been one of my main concerns as a sex educator. An impasse over oral sex, as over any core sexual practice of great importance to the success of an erotic relationship, must be resolved in one of two ways: Either the relationship is fated to fail over this deadlock and both partners should resume their searches for more compatible mates or a compromise must be reached.

In other words, this might be a situation where you would be wise to do unto another as you would have done unto you. While a significant group of people dislikes performing oral sex, a far smaller group dislikes receiving it. If the price of a happy pussy eager to be fucked is

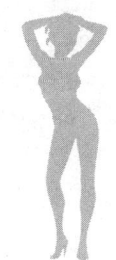

overcoming a mild resistance to showing it a happy face first, I suggest you consider where your own best interests lie and make the necessary internal adjustments. Believe me, I'll offer similar advice on the subject of fellatio in due course. Some things we love to learn; other things we learn to love.

There are women who don't like receiving cunnilingus, for whatever reason, preferring other forms of foreplay. As with the example cited above, if her partner really likes cunnilingus, she's well advised to find a way to enjoy her partner's honest pleasure and delight in her body. By seeing herself through her partner's eyes, she may come to a new level of self-acceptance, finally able to be her bad self.

Know Your Objective

Cunnilingus is not a competitive sport. It has no single goal but rather a multiplicity of purposes. For some women, cunnilingus leads to orgasms as nothing else can. For others, it's a vital element of foreplay, without which penetrative intercourse is essentially a labor of love. While recent writings on the subject of female sexuality have tended to deemphasize intercourse as a source of orgasmic pleasure and to stress external, clitoral stimulation as the only road to sexual satisfaction, there are still many women for whom penetration is the main event and oral sex is simply a pleasant distraction between erections. Many women can orgasm from both cunnilingus and intercourse, and these are lucky ladies, indeed. Some men are highly aroused by the intimate contact of mouth on vulva. Others practice cunnilingus as a form of worship, meant to convey a strong desire to please and appreciation for the opportunity to do so. All these motivations are equally legitimate and worthy of respect.

At its finest, oral sex raises the level of stimulation and intensity in a stair-step fashion: periods of fast-paced sucking interspersed with languid plateaus of slow munching that protract the pleasure of the total experience for as long as desired. Keep in mind that you don't "give" your partner orgasms; you can only offer your assistance through your attention to her desires. It may take months of practice before she can come from oral sex. Don't rush this part, and don't worry if it never happens. The goal is always easy, mutual pleasure. The exact form that pleasure takes is a discovery you'll make along the way.

Half as Fast, Twice as Long

Though I never pass up the opportunity to point out the basic similarities between men and women when it comes to sex, there are always a few differences worthy of note. When it comes to oral sex, men are more likely to derive the greatest benefit from firm, rapid stimulation after an initial period of protracted teasing. Women need less focused intensity spread out over a larger area for a longer period of time. Ideally, cunnilingus will be equally pleasurable to both partners, and neither will feel a need to rush it to some kind of conclusion, either from a need to get on to other things, a lack of enthusiasm for the ac-

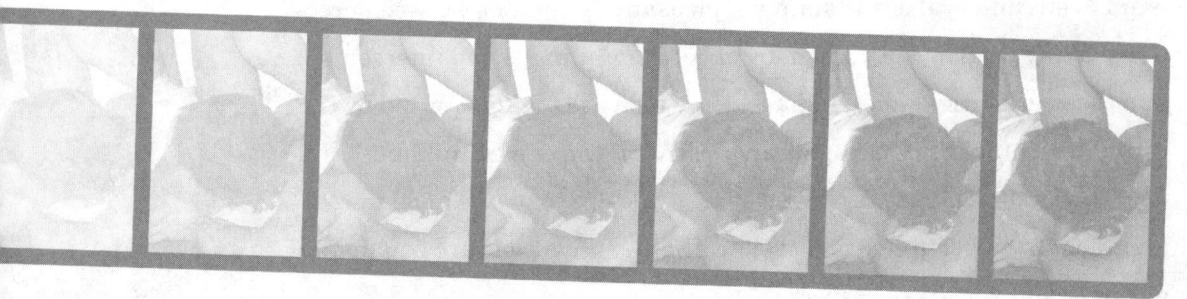

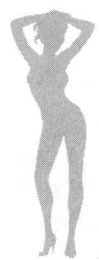

tivity itself, or guilt about being the recipient of a partner's attentions. That a dating couple would linger over a nice dinner for two hours and then accept a mere three minutes of pussy eating for dessert strikes me as poor prioritizing. Whatever you hope to achieve with cunnilingus— a chain reaction of multiple orgasms that rock the foundations of the house or a state of urgent need that precedes an intense coupling— take your time. Some things in life are simply too good to rush.

HOT LICKS

1 • *If you're a guy, shave first.* Very few women masturbate with sandpaper.

2 • *If you're a girl, whether you shave or not, make sure you're clean enough down there* that you wouldn't mind using your own tongue if it would reach that far.

3 • *Flicking sucks.* Sucking rocks.

4 • *It's okay to talk with your mouth full.* If you want to know if you're doing it right, ask her.

5 • *Take your time.* You'll be glad you did.

6 • *A little biting goes a long way.* Keep the tooth action light and brief.

7 • *Girls, let your appreciation show.* I've never yet met a man who didn't like the feel of a woman's legs wrapped around his shoulders.

8 • *Mix it up.* Try some cunnilingus, then some sex, some more cunnilingus, some more sex, etc. This will keep her nicely revved up while you work your way into that new position you want to try.

LINGUAL LAPSES

1 • *Don't fall prey to pussy fever.* I know you're excited to be there and all, but never forget that it's attached to a real person. The rest of her needs attention from time to time.

2 • *Do NOT trace the alphabet on her clit,* write her name with your tongue, or attempt other fancy-schmancy tricks. Grab a mouthful and suck.

3 • *Avoid pretending to be a hummingbird.* Having the fastest tongue in the West won't help you here, partner. Let her set the rhythm with her hip movements.

4 • *No biting.* A bit of tooth friction in the right place at the right time can be yummy, but, unlike dicks, clits generally don't like being used as chew toys.

5 • *Don't do it by the numbers.* Believe me, we can tell when you're going down the checklist.

6 • *Don't set time limits.* Looking at your watch and deciding she's had enough tells her just how much you care about her pleasure.

7 • *When something is working, don't interrupt.* If she's rocking her hips and moaning, that's a signal for you to keep right on doing whatever it is you're doing now.

8 • *Don't be afraid to use your hands or hers.* Let her show you where her secret treasures are hidden. She knows the terrain better than you do.

Chapter 7

FELLATIO:
MAKING HIS KNOB THROB

ellatio was the first sex skill I perfected, and it hasn't failed me yet. Being so close to a man's most tender parts never ceases to thrill me. I find penises and scrotums charming and sweet, responding to stimulation with an irrepressible honesty that's consistently inspiring. Face-to-face with a penis, I always know where we both stand, even if I happen to be on my knees.

It still amazes me that after so many years of open discussion of this elementary and primal sexual activity, it's still the source of so much discord and disappointment in the lives of so many couples. I know the vast majority of men desire it, as they never hesitate to tell me, and I like to think that most women in heterosexual relationships enjoy it, too. And yet I still hear laments from men whose partners are reluctant fellatrices at best and from women who continue to feel pressured to engage in an act they find degrading or disgusting.

While I try not to be judgmental and prefer to hope that there's somebody out there for everyone, I must candidly admit that, were I a man, I wouldn't have a long-term sex partner who wouldn't suck my cock with sincere enthusiasm. As a woman, I certainly wouldn't entertain for a moment the idea of mating with a man who took no pleasure in eagerly applying his mouth to my pussy. In my view, neither a man nor a woman can be considered an accomplished lover without a basic oral skill set and a willingness to deploy it generously. A sexologist friend of mine believes that if all wives and girlfriends cultivated a love of fellatio and engaged in it regularly, visits to sex professionals would drop off by upward of 90 percent, effective immediately. So girls, unless you want someone like me as your competition, get ready to suck it up, literally.

Fellatio isn't a task to be endured for the benefit of another. It's a selfish pleasure all its own. Your enjoyment of it, more than any specific technique I'll describe, will determine how effectively you and your man connect in this uniquely human fashion. When you have a man by the balls, as the saying goes, his heart and mind will follow, so your intentions must be good.

An eager willingness to suck cock confers much power on the giver, who controls the pacing, atmosphere, and specific physical elements of the experience. If your guy is shy, you can inspire him to show you a really good time. If he's too frisky, you can slow him down by insisting that he lie back and take it like a man. If he's not in the mood and you are, a good blow job can be very persuasive. If you're not in the mood and he is, you can get yourself there by indulging your taste for man flesh. Knowing that your partner is already having fun is an unfailing

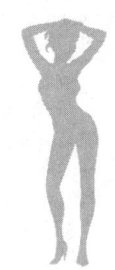

confidence builder. In short, there's a blow job for every occasion and for every need, and the fellatrix determines the outcome. Though some women, myself included, enjoy the service aspect of oral worship, fellatio empowers women more than any other penetrative sex act. This truth has been reinforced throughout human history and continues to be every day.

Fellatio, however, is not an Olympic event. You needn't be able to swallow a whole cucumber to feel confident, relaxed, and sure of your skills. What you do need is a real desire. If you want to be known as a gal who gives monster skull, only passion can make it happen. I can teach you how to do it, but it's up to you to learn to love it. For starters, let's get down there and have a good look at what's on the bill of fare.

Meeting Dick

To become truly adept at fellatio, you must love, love, love men and, by extension, their penises. If you treat them like the Loch Ness monster, that's about how often you can expect them to put in an appearance. Having seen quite a few of them up close, I can state with conviction that no two are alike, that each has its charms, and that I've never met one that didn't reflect the personality of its owner in some way. If you like the man enough to have sex with him, his intimate anatomy should attract rather than repel you. If that's not the case, you may be with an inappropriate partner who fails to appeal to you in other ways as well. There is nothing inherently dirty or distasteful about oral contact with a penis, including the fact that a man urinates out of it. Our own reproductive and excretory organs also exist in close proximity. Within the requirements of rudimentary personal hygiene—a must for both genders when it comes to sex, especially of the oral persuasion—

there is nothing about a man's cock and balls that's intrinsically unappetizing.

For all their quirks, penises present pretty much the same zones of opportunity when it comes to oral sex. Viewing a man's package from its level, one first encounters his penis, resting on top of his testicles. If he is uncircumcised, the glans is plainly visible. Depending on the circumstances (in an unheated stable, for example), the glans may be the only part of his penis visible at that moment. A flaccid penis averages between two and five inches long, though obviously I've met men whose equipment falls outside those specs. They are an occupational hazard of my line of work. Though I have encountered women who prefer the supersize model, I still regard penile size as primarily a male preoccupation. Normal is good, and most of us prefer it as a steady diet, however consumed.

If he's not circumcised ("natural" or "uncut," in porn slang), his foreskin will cover the glans, and his penis will look like something out of classical art. As with a woman's labia, a foreskin provides just the right amount of protection and lubrication for casual masturbation. If you find your partner is uncut, pull the skin up over the head of his cock and squeeze it together. Gently lick, suck, nibble, and explore the delicate folds. In moments like these, do to his foreskin what you like to have done to your inner lips. As you pull the skin up and loose, sneak your tongue in between the glans and head. Pay attention to what makes his cock swell and throb in your hand. When an uncircumcised man is aroused, his penis will expand and his foreskin will retract, exposing the head. Keep it that way before putting on a condom.

The glans may be fat, round, wide, narrow, blunt, or pointy. When aroused, it may be either bigger in circumference than the shaft itself or smaller. The glans is flared on top, making an effective spot to rub

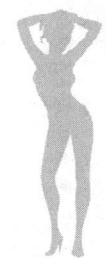

with a fist or lip-covered teeth. At the tip is the opening to the urethra, and beneath that is the frenum, the most sensitive spot on a penis, where the head meets the shaft. Along with the shaft, the glans also fills with blood when he's aroused and becomes springier in texture. Some are so big I can't get them into my mouth very well without scraping them, and some fit all the way back to my tonsils effortlessly. It's going to swell in your mouth either way. Take that as a compliment.

The shaft, when soft, may be pulled up short and tight or hang down low and loose. Some men are "showers" and some are "growers," so it's nearly impossible to predict the size of a man's erection by looking at his resting penis. When he's hard, a guy's penis may be fat, thin, long, short, curved, bent, smooth, veiny, wedge-shaped, knob-shaped, blunt, or pointed. One of my favorites of all time was thinner at the base and tip and fatter in the middle. *Umm,* dreamy!

The base of the cock is the best place to get a grip before putting your oral skills to work. Wrap your hand around it and squeeze. As with squeezing a balloon, you'll produce a bulge at the head. Now relax your grip, let him contract his muscles, and repeat this little exercise a couple of times. Feel his reflexive squeeze and trace a spit-wet fingertip over the glans or frenum while you watch his reaction. Nice, huh? It will react even more happily to the same action from your tongue.

Hanging down behind the penis is the scrotum, which contains the testicles. Some men's balls are always on the high, tight side, even when exposed to warm environments, and some men's are always on the low, dangly side, even in the cold, but most scrotums pull up when it's cold or when their owners are about to come, and hang low when their owners are relaxed and warm. Balls come in many sizes, from two to a mouth all the way to not even one fits. Some guys like pressure on their balls; some don't. When you're down there, reach up to fondle them, pulling on the skin between them, rubbing the bulb of his penis, making his balls swing. Bring one testicle into your mouth and tilt your head back slightly as you pull his cock up toward his head. Play with your pussy while you use your mouth and other hand on him. It's hot to watch and reminds you that this is for the both of you.

By now, you've examined the goods and perhaps sampled them a bit. From here on, attitude and action will need to work in concert to produce the results that will cause everybody at the office to wonder what he's smiling about the next day. How you feel about what you do is the single most important factor determining how what you do will feel.

Getting into the Proper Headspace

As with any sex skill, your emotional state is easily 60 percent of the game, and that part is mainly your responsibility, assuming you're with a partner you trust and desire (and if you're not, you can just skip this part and send out for Chinese food). Women have widely differing reactions to the notion of sucking dick. Some, like me, are enthusiastic and always have been, even when we weren't very experienced at it. Some would like to get good at it but are hampered by social conditioning they haven't yet overcome. Others don't like the idea much but want to satisfy their lovers and are willing to bypass a bit of internal resistance for a worthwhile cause. A small, but persistent, percentage of the female population is just not having any part of it, no how, no way, no matter what. The first group needs no encouragement from me, and the last group doesn't want my help at all, so I'll address my comments on mind-set to the two middle groups.

As I mentioned earlier, when social conditioning gets in the way of intimate happiness, a choice must be faced: Get beyond the condition-

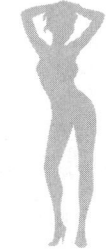

ing and accept pleasure and intimacy or continue to avoid the behavior and forgo the opportunity to discover your natural response to it. Which will it be? Will you listen to the disapproving voices of the past still rattling around your brain, or will you take a minute to figure out how you came to resist such an elemental source of satisfaction and get over yourself? I've sucked a lot of cock and never once has the earth opened up to swallow me, a thunderbolt from heaven blasted me to smithereens, or a phone call from my mother gotten in the way.

Some women shy away from fellatio because they feel awkward and don't want to appear clumsy, inexperienced, or inhibited. It's easy to be intimidated by the expectations that popular culture layers on top of whatever insecurities you may own. This anxiety can be overcome by practicing the simple, physical skill set I'll get to soon. Other women may hold back out of a common, though rarely justified, fear that men will think less of them or consider them only "one of those sluts who suck dick." Any man so conflicted as to receive a blow job from a woman and then dump on her for giving it doesn't deserve a lover and should be replaced by someone who does. A woman may have had one or more unpleasant experiences with fellatio with unsuitable partners that still haunt her. If any of the above describes your feelings, you can use the penis at your disposal to dispel them.

Nurse Nina says: "Genitals are not unsanitary." Like any other body part, when freshly washed with hot water and a nice mild soap, they smell and taste like human skin, the kind with which you, too, are upholstered. Here, your partner can help out by presenting you with appetizing prospects. It will serve his cause if he trims his pubic hair and/or shaves his scrotum, since a lot of women find the "hairy nut sac" particularly off-putting. Even waxing has caught on with some men, to the gratitude of the women in their lives, who can empathize with the commitment implied. You may still have reservations, but at least you've got your face near something clean and smooth.

While some men will abuse the privilege of having a dick in a woman's mouth, most do so only out of overeagerness and a lack of experience. They will generally respond to clear verbal and physical signals setting limits for the role they're to play as recipients of a special gift. There need not, and should not, be any power struggle over who initiates what. He may propose, but it's up to you to dispose. It's okay to disclose your hesitations and to proceed at a pace that feels natural. There is no objective standard of excellence to which you need aspire, only the generation of sensations you both enjoy. If you have the ambition to suck cock like a porn star, you'll eventually learn how, but in the meantime you can both enjoy a process of discovery that need never be less than pleasant in any way.

The proper headspace for approaching cock sucking is one of trust and acceptance, not in the certainty of a particular result but rather in the mutual respect that makes the process of discovery itself pleasurable. This is every bit as true for men as it is for women. There is an art to giving an excellent blow job and an art to receiving one. A man who allows himself to be entertained, who makes eye contact, who touches his partner's hair, face, and breasts pleasingly while she works her magic does more than just make her feel appreciated. He participates in the pleasure just as fully as she does.

It May Be a Job, but It's Not All Work

For a serious blow job, get comfortable. If you're kneeling on the floor while he sits, make sure that your knees are cushioned, since damage to the cartilage is cumulative, and that he's sitting on a towel

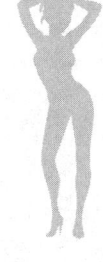

to protect the furniture. He should be naked or nearly so. You'll need lube, water, and a towel or baby wipes nearby. Taking his stuff in your hands, play with it, lifting, twisting, juggling, etc., while you look up at him flirtatiously. Nothing, and I mean no thing, is sexier to a guy than seeing a happy, willing woman on her knees in front of him. Let him play with your hair, say sweet things, and stroke your face as you tell him whatever is true: "You feel so good"; "I'm looking forward to this!" "*Ooh,* you're getting harder"; "It's okay/not okay to pull my hair," etc. If you're dressed to enhance and display your cleavage, double points for you for understanding that men are very visual. Use that power for good, not evil, and show yourself a fine time along with his. You're being adorable; let him adore you.

There are three basic ways to give head. You can: (1) remain in control at all times, teasing him as you please while he relaxes and enjoys the show; (2) get into the receptive mode, letting his responses guide your movements; (3) and/or trade off initiatives, taking turns at the wheel. Until I know someone pretty well, I always start with the first approach. Most men are more than content to let me take the lead. Once you acquire the confidence that practice confers, however you play out the dynamics of a particular situation, you'll communicate that confidence to your partner. Without fail, if you're enjoying yourself, so will he, and the evidence will be impossible to overlook.

If you start lying on a bed, try pressing your face against the bulb of his cock until you're breathing together and he's twitching. Hard or soft, pull his cock up and nuzzle his balls apart. Plant a warm, deep, slow kiss on the space between them. Squeeze his cock (palm down will be most ergonomic) as you pull it while you do little press-release moves with your mouth. Hold your face still and stroke the full length of his cock, releasing when you come to the tip. Fellatio is an acquired pleasure, so take your time sampling it. Suck, lick, nibble, squeeze, stroke, even bite (after you ask!) his cock and balls, letting yourself sink into the dreamy, languid space of unhurried enjoyment.

If you're on your knees, hold his balls in both hands and bury your face in them as you would a bouquet of flowers. Feel his balls roll around in your hand, notice how soft the skin is, how his hard-or-not cock feels on your cheek. Be very still, and feel how his balls move on their own, controlled by a subconscious force. His cock may start to stir against your cheek. If so, take as much of it in your mouth as you can, press down with your mouth to create a little suction, and pull it out as far as you can before releasing it again. Soft cocks can be fun to play with too. Nuzzle your face in his groin. If he's standing, get underneath him and press your face into his balls, letting them drape themselves over you as you feel his bulb twitch. If you're lucky, there will be just enough man scent to be a turn-on.

The skin of a cock is velvety soft. Suck and nibble on it. The frenum sticks out a bit. Give it some attention as well. Put him in your mouth and suck the fleshy softness until he swells so much he doesn't fit. When he's hard, bite slowly and delicately into the head until you feel that unmistakable quiver, then release quickly and take all of it in your mouth. Use his cock to rub and stimulate your mouth, inspiring hot and thrilling fantasies to make you juicer and wetter. It's fun to be in control, to feel so sexy and desirable. Don't short-change yourself here.

Time to focus your attentions on some serious pleasure giving. Keeping one hand cupped on the bulb, work his cock with the other in long, twisty strokes. It feels good when you use both hands, twisting them in opposition to each other as you slide up and down the shaft. Add your mouth, going down as far as you can as you loosen your grip, and then holding tight while pulling up with your mouth and hand. Use your lips

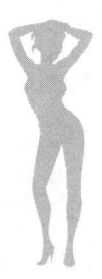

to cover your teeth while you stroke him in and out. When you feel him getting close, or he tells you that he is, change the rhythm to back him off, switching to a lighter or slower touch. It's a wonderful power rush to keep a guy on the edge of coming for as long as you like. Both of you have to have good discipline, but it's a blast to drive him wild with pleasure.

In taking control in this fashion, you also take responsibility for respecting your partner's limits. Teasing is great, but there is a point of diminishing returns. Make note of the things your partner likes best and, well before frustration and fading arousal set in, settle on a dependable routine of identified favorites. Also be aware that lengthy, focused stimulation, particularly at the opening of the glans, can produce an unpleasant hypersensitivity he may be reluctant to acknowledge for fear of seeming ungrateful.

There's nothing wrong with letting him lead if that's what you both prefer. Once he's in your mouth, wrap one or both hands around his cock. This will act as a "bumper" to prevent an accidental thrust from going too deep and triggering your gag reflex. There are no fancy tongue tricks to do here, or nibbles or nuzzles. Just tighten your mouth and hands on the out-stroke, then loosen both on the in-stroke. His hands on your head create an emotional connection and help him guide his thrusts. Though society doesn't recognize it properly, there is also power in receptivity. Try matching him stroke for stroke or just lolling back and allowing him to fuck your face.

You only need let him go as deep as you find comfortable. Much too much has been made of the whole "deep throat" thing. The most responsive parts of the penis are nearest the end and along the first quarter of the shaft. Cock swallowing can be an erotic treat for those whose parts fit together correctly to make it possible, but it's by no means necessary for a lovely oral-sex session.

I know some women who seem to have been born without gag reflexes, allowing them to get all sorts of things down their throats, but the rest of us have them for a reason: It's lifesaving. I've devised an alternative to tossing my cookies in his lap that no man has objected to yet, something I've labeled "snarffling." This entails getting his cock as far back into my mouth as I comfortably can, then pushing forward a half inch or so, until my gag reflex is triggered just a little bit. The involuntary constriction of my muscles around his cock is dramatic and exciting and demonstrates that I'm trying my darndest to get it all in there. I can tolerate three almost-gags in a row before I have to pull him out and return to my regular blow job. The vagus nerve stimulated by this move will also trigger a tear or two from you, sweet proof of your determination.

Most often, you'll trade off control of the action. You can get him going, then sit back and have him feed his dick to you. You can tease him by popping his cock in and out of your mouth, or he can tease you by popping his cock in and out of your mouth, in between slapping it gently (or not) against your lips or rubbing it on your face. Between the right two people, this is a powerful, perfectly respectful expression of arousal. In short, get playful with it. That's the atmosphere in which the best oral sex will predictably occur.

Taking in the Surrounding Sights

Specifically, I'm talking about his balls, bulb, and butt. We've already seen how important stimulation of the bulb is to his pleasure. Scrotums often enjoy being pulled, stretched, bitten, twisted, scratched, and tickled. What he'll like best will depend on whether his sac is low, loose, and thin or tight, thick, and wrinkled. Testicles may re-

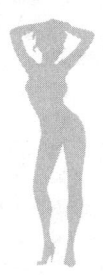

spond favorably to being gently pulled into the mouth and popped out again. When playing with them, keep in mind that the tender, potentially painful region of the testicle is the bumpy part at the top end. This is the *epididymis,* where mature sperm are stored, waiting for the "go" signal. If you avoid the epididymis, testicles can take a fair amount of pressure. Let his response guide you, as some men really like testicular manipulation, whereas others are scared to death of it.

More and more men are tuning in to the pleasure of anal play, and the best place to start is with external stimulation, using fingers or mouths. There will be a complete discussion about anal pleasure and hygiene in our subsequent exploration of anal sex. Butt play requires delicate negotiation for parties of either gender. To start out, make a deal and stick to it: If he'll let you play with the outside of his butt, you won't do anything invasive without further deliberation. Licking, tickling, stretching, and massaging the anal ring are all very pleasurable and perfectly sanitary. If you can, while he's in your mouth, reach around and grab his butt cheeks and massage them. This stretches his anus and makes him aware of it. He'll probably fuck your face a little more passionately as well.

Imaginative Extras

Some men, for reasons unknown to me, really like a cold sensation on their balls or cock. It's difficult to improve on an enthusiastic hand-and-mouth combo, but it's worth a try to put some ice by the bed before you start. When you've got him going, grab a few ice chips and put them in your mouth, then put your mouth around his cock. It will startle him, certainly, but after a second or two, he should be able to tell you if he likes it or not. Failed experiments need not be repeated.

I'm generally not a fan of combining food with sex, preferring the taste of clean skin, but if it helps get things going to put a bit of whipped cream or chocolate syrup on his cock, there's no reason not to. It's important to make sure that all such condiments are cleaned off before fucking, as sugar-based foodstuffs don't interact well with the chemistry of pussies.

To spit or to swallow? That is the question we all must face. Since I don't like the taste of semen (it's alkaline, to neutralize the acidity of the vagina for sperm), if a man comes in my mouth I generally swallow. Why? By the time he's done coming, his cum is gone instead of remaining to annoy you. You can always have a glass of soda next to the bed to cover the taste, if you prefer.

If you're just not ready for oral ejaculation, when he tells you he's close, pull him out of your mouth and either one of you can jerk him to a finish on your boobs or, for a real "porno" climax, on your mouth or cheek. (Avoid the eyes—*ouch!*) Both men and women have been mercilessly guilt-tripped about the political implications of this common behavior, from which both can derive great satisfaction under the right conditions. You're grown-ups and nobody's watching. Make whatever kind of mess you both like. You give each other and yourselves permission. No other votes will be counted.

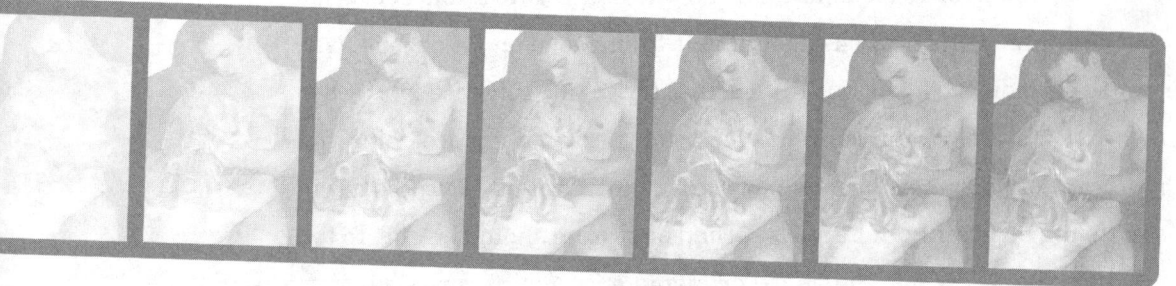

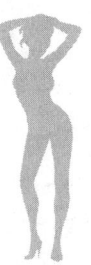

BLOW-JOB BASICS

1 • *Enthusiasm is more important than technique.* The more you like what you're doing, the more he'll like it, too.

2 • *Start slow but be prepared to speed up at the end.* A surprising degree of friction is often needed to produce the desired finale.

3 • *Guys, do your part.* By word, gesture, and expression, let us know our labors are appreciated.

4 • *Women are beautiful with cocks in their mouths.* Position your body to give him a nice view, and don't be afraid to make eye contact.

5 • *You get no points for being a neat eater.* Biology is untidy, and that's how it's meant to be.

6 • *It's okay to make some noise.*

7 • *Learning to breathe through your nose with a rigid object sliding in and out of your mouth takes practice.* A small dildo makes a handy training aid.

8 • *Know where it's all going to end.* If you're spooling up for a hot fuck, linger an extra moment before moving on. If you're sucking to completion, agree on the drop zone in advance.

BLOW-JOB BLUNDERS

1 • *Careful with those teeth.* They're designed to cut meat.

2 • *Don't be shy.* Firm pressure shows confidence and feels better to you.

3 • *Do not neglect the outlying areas.* Lingering too long on one spot can get old in a hurry.

4 • *Boys, no grabbing her head and thrusting deeply into her mouth without prior permission.* It could be dangerous.

5 • *Avoid changing the cadence when he's close to finally coming.* When it's time for the pop, find the best rhythm and stick with it to the end.

6 • *Lose the hidden agendas.* Hoping to trade a long-withheld BJ for something in a baby-blue box courts well-deserved disappointment.

7 • *Failure to give proper warning is grounds for subsequent refusal.* When the explosion is imminent, a gentleman owes a lady the choice of where to receive the blast.

Chapter 8

MAKING LOVE TO WOMEN: PUSHING HER BUTTONS

Now you're in bed, naked, with your lovely lady, and she's in receptive mode, ready to be taken for a ride. What do you do? Whatever you do, take it slow. Eventually, if she's really going to go the distance with you, she'll make that clear. Never forget that consent is an ongoing process and she can quit whenever she wants with no static from you. The law says this, and so do I. Meantime, the more kissing, hugging, and rolling around you do, the better. While this chapter is addressed to men, smart women will want to give it plenty of attention in the hopes of heightening their own pleasure and that of their partner. We want to know how your body feels all over, not just in the naughty bits, before we close the deal. Hug her, then slowly, steadily, equally, hug tighter and tighter, legs included. It's important to keep it equal; your strength-under-control is very sexy. Provide just enough resistance to get her panting, then release the pressure.

Looking deep into her eyes is nice, but some of your best work needs to come standing from behind. Try wrapping an arm around her upper arms, gently pulling them together. This yogic spine loosener has the added benefits of arching her back toward you, thrusting out her breasts and making it easy for her head to fall back against your shoulder. She's exposed, relaxed, and waiting. Kiss and nibble on her ear or neck while your free hand runs firmly up and down her body, squeezing her tits, stroking her face, and gently grasping her neck. If you're in front of a mirror, tell her to look at how hot she is. Stroke her body, and your hand will naturally end up at her vulva at about the same time she cradles your balls and the bulb of your penis in one hand, your cock in the other.

Just as there are all shapes and sizes of penises and scrotums, so, too, is there a great variety of pussy types. Some are wide, shallow V's, with tidy lips and meaty fat pads over the pubic bone. Grab that pad, and your fingertip will naturally be guided to the top of her cleft. Lifting her mound will pull the cleft up. This will masturbate her with exquisite delicacy. Others have narrower V's and bonier architecture, with no perceptible upholstery over the frame. Some clits are deeply hidden, whereas the hoods of other clits are clearly visible even without pulling the labia apart. Some women have meaty lips that hang down from the pubic bone, and others seem to have no extra flesh to speak of, merely little slits between their legs. Different massage and manipulation techniques work best with different types of vulvas. Simple trial and error will quickly reveal which methods are most effective with your particular partner.

If you're lying between her legs in such a manner that she can grind against your abdomen, start there as you kiss her and play with her

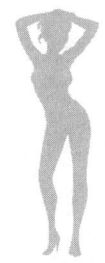

breasts. These lead-ins, as we established in the chapter on foreplay, aren't means to an end; they are part of the total process that awakens nerve endings and stirs the imagination. Soon enough, if you both display the proper mix of confidence and respectful restraint, she'll crave direct attention to her pussy. Clean, smooth hands and short, well-kept nails are musts for what follows. Personally, I favor latex exam gloves (now available in sexy black latex on the Net) for internal stimulation of any sort, just to avoid the perils of ragged cuticles and rough patches.

I know that pussies can seem very intimidating, unknowable or unreadable at first glance, but their secrets aren't that closely held. The pussy of a woman who is happy to be in bed with you gives clear and unambiguous signals, once you know what to look for. More accurately, it's a matter of knowing what to feel for, since it's the subtle, internal movements of her muscles that tell the tale. While still kissing and making as much full-body contact as possible, place your hand over her vulva and squeeze. The heel of your hand will force her clit toward your fingers, which feels as good as when you grab your dickhead and give it a pull. Or a genital first contact can entail cupping her pubic bone from above as you put your thumb and forefinger on one side of her vulva and your other fingers on the other side, squeezing them together, trapping her clit between your fingers. At that point, all you have to do is kiss her as she masturbates with your hand. You don't have to "do" anything else. You can alternate cupping the pubic bone with pinching her lips to trap her clit between your thumb and fingers. Do not confuse her clit with the Fire Rockets button on a video game. Rapid, repeated motion produces irritation rather than ignition. If there's going to be any frantic friction at the eventual point of climax, leave that to her.

For this next move, you'll want a few drops of lube to put on her vestibule (not to be confused with her foyer, lest you end up in court over a slip-and-fall incident). Place your thumb on one side of the base of her clit at the pubic bone, between the inner and outer lips, and your middle or ring finger on the other side of her shaft, also between the inner and outer lips. Your forefinger (or forefinger and middle finger) will naturally land on the underside of her clit. With very small motions, make like you're taking a pinch from a pile of salt. Do this rhythmically, with your wrist loose, about one pinch per second, and you'll be jilling her off more effectively than any attempt to emulate an electric vibrator. Just imagine the move you use on yourself when you masturbate. Picture that same stroke if your cock was two inches shorter, four inches shorter, so short it's only a nub. Keep this in mind, and she'll find you brilliant.

You know how you place your fingers on your frenum with your thumb on top of your cock when you're masturbating? You know those subtle movements you make right down the center of your shaft, the little tickling ones, barely moving your fingers at all? News flash: Those same moves work for her. Lube up her pussy, paying special attention to the outer surfaces. Lying next to her, reach over and put your forefinger (or, if your hands are big, your middle finger) on the shaft of her clit, between her inner and outer lips where it meets the pubic bone. Keeping them close together, line up your other fingers, placing them under the head of her clit. Do those same short strokes that you like on your frenum, only even smaller if you can.

Try keeping your fingers in place without moving them at all. Just press gently but firmly down on her pubic bone while pushing her shaft to one side. You may not feel like you're doing much, but her breathing and undulating will provide the needed friction. Think of the shaft of her clit as a guitar string and her pubic bone as the fret, and "play" her. The smallest motions transmit a great deal of sensation. You'll mainly be supplying the pressure while she'll be managing the moves. If she's

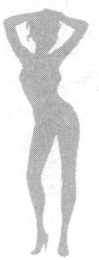

grabbing your cock at this time, you can mirror your touches on each other, building heat and intimacy in a gradual crescendo.

As your partner gets more excited, she may start working herself against your hand with surprising intensity. No worries: Vulvas are remarkably sturdy and like to be handled firmly, providing the handler knows what he's doing. Once she's fully aroused, "grab" her pussy quite firmly, IF you know where to place your hand. If the heel of your hand makes contact at exactly the right spot on her pubic bone, automatically wrapping your fingers to cup her lips as you rub her clit, you're literally in the groove. If you dig your fingernails into her tender flesh and pull abruptly, she'll snap out of the mood instantly, which could be a bad thing if she happens to have your nuts in her grip at the time.

The secret to always getting these details right is never to let your arousal take you so far into your own body that you no longer pay proper attention to hers. No matter how hot you get, how hard, how excited, she must always feel that you're reading her and paying attention. If you frighten or annoy her, it's all over. In order to get her to turn off her brain and settle into her body, it must know, at the cellular level, that it's safe. I'm a very mental person, and it's hard for me to let go and just do it. I do, however, trust my body not to steer me wrong. I'll let a man touch me for as long as he makes me feel good, but no longer. The better he tunes into me, the longer he gets to play. It's a win-win situation. How you'll learn to stay focused during this process is up to you, and there are books in the Bibliography that may be helpful.

Reading Her Signals

Here's a little trick for keeping you both involved when it's time to move on to cunnilingus: Tilt her slightly up onto one hip, lube the arch of the foot that's on the bed (her left foot if she's on her left hip, etc.), and arrange your bodies so that you can rub your cock and balls on it while you eat and massage her pussy. The foot is full of nerves and very sensitive, so it's lovely for her, unless she's ticklish beyond belief, in which case give it up at the first giggle. It also feels a lot better on your cock than humping rough sheets. Within a few minutes, you'll want to add internal massage, a vital prelude to the effective insertion of larger body parts. Keep in mind that fingers and cocks are not interchangeable, and each has its place in the scheme of pussy pleasuring. When using your fingers, take advantage of what they can do that cocks can't: articulate. Fingers can probe and prod every secret inch of a woman's insides, tickling her G-spot or finding that special hot zone in her *lateral fornix* that drives her crazy (I told you these directions would come in handy!).

Women's internal geographies are unique, and fingers can investigate them in ways that cocks can't. Make a "V for Victory" sign (or a peace sign if you're of a certain generation) and bend the fingers into a slight hook. When you slip those two fingers into her, don't try to fuck her with them as you would with your cock. Two slender digits simply aren't meaty enough to do anything for her, no matter how hard she squeezes her pelvic muscles, and nothing is more annoying than a guy copying some porn video by frantically frigging. It looks lame in pictures, and it feels even more so in real life.

Calm down, slow down, and let yourself get lost in the wonder that is pussy. Lube up two fingers. Turn them pads down and slide them in to about the second knuckle. Keeping them flat, rub in little circles as you press against the muscle. Note how her pussy tenses and relaxes against your fingers. When it feels right, and using more lube as needed, slide your fingers all the way back until your remaining knuckles press firmly

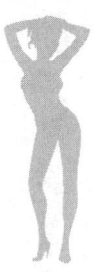

against her vulva and clit. Press down against the muscle for a count of four, gently stretching the opening of her pussy. Press and relax, press and relax, and see how she responds. If nothing much seems to be happening, press more firmly but not roughly. The goal here is to elicit involuntary sounds of pleasure, to help her sink more deeply into the moment.

Next, sweep your fingers from about the three o'clock position to the nine o'clock position and notice exactly which location generates her deepest, most excited moans. You'll need to know this when you're fucking her, as she'll like your cock in that spot as well. While every woman is different, for some reason eight o'clock seems a consistent favorite, statistically speaking. Now, with your fingers all the way in and facing down, spread them apart (that "V for Victory" move again) at about the four and seven o'clock positions. Bend your fingers and pull your hand toward you an inch or three, applying pressure to her internal muscles. Pulling and releasing repeatedly should elicit happy, deeply relaxed verbalizations.

Now that you've made a favorable first impression, simply arch your wrist up as you push forward a bit, directing your fingertips toward her butt and your knuckles onto her clit, and then flatten it, pulling your hand out slightly. On the in-stroke, s-l-o-w-l-y push very firmly, enough to move her whole body away from you, then release the pressure on the out-stroke. Your hand won't actually travel very far, but you'll be moving her internal muscles and, in fact, her whole body. This sets up the beat for actual intercourse, mobilizing her pelvis for more strenuous activities to follow. Mix up deep pushing, side-to-side sweeping, forked-finger pulling, and bent-wrist pressure with any other tickling that elicits a favorable response, but don't change too quickly from one type of manipulation to the next.

To really get into the groove, there has to *be* one, so stay with a sensation that seems to be doing it for her. The man who can contain his own rising excitement and continue revving her up to speed will be rewarded. Indulge your voyeurism. A woman growing increasingly aroused by your skilled efforts is a beautiful sight to behold. As desired, any of these moves can be accompanied by pinching her clit in that delicious manner or with her masturbating. Don't be afraid to let her help you out; this isn't your show or hers, but rather a joint production.

You'll need some different strokes to stimulate the G-spot. Here, fingers can be either flat or crooked, depending on whether diffuse or direct sensation is desired. Some women prefer their G-spots rubbed, whereas others require a pointed poke, almost hooking the pubic bone. Be patient during some trial-and-error experimentation. If an in-and-out sensation is desired, point your fingers almost toward the ceiling, knuckles pressed firmly on the *fourchette*. They won't penetrate into her pussy more than two inches, and they don't need to. The combination of the entry being rubbed, pressed, and stretched (remember, the opening to the vagina is friction sensitive and the back of the pussy is pressure sensitive) and the G-spot being stimulated is simply fabulous. Combine the vulva-clit pinch with the *fourchette*-push/G-spot tickle. You should feel her pussy practically pulsate. If you're limber, you can also combine pussy eating with the deep finger massage, a sure thing when done properly.

When friction is called for, three fingers will usually do it, with your third and first fingers placed in front of your middle finger: yet another bastardized version of the Scout salute. The trick here (in addition to proper lubrication, of course) is combining the in-and-out movement with rotation of the wrist, adding an extra zing to the friction. As the heat builds, the tensing/relaxing of her muscles will be increasingly obvious. In general, when her pussy tenses up, keep the strokes shallow,

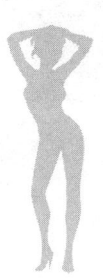

short, and light. When she relaxes, make the strokes firmer, longer, and deeper. You'll feel her pussy suck your fingers in and push them out. Add more fingers as are welcome. Her pussy can change up every five strokes, so stay focused. If you're like me, it's never a chore.

Women who climax easily from penetration may go over the edge from these activities alone, generally signaling the beginning of a mighty fine evening. If she starts to come while you're still in the hands-on (or, more correctly, hands-in) phase, with or without vibrator assistance, do not change whatever it is you're doing or she'll lose her momentum. No matter how excited you are, or how furiously you'd love to frig her over the edge, remain aware and in control. Unless she says "Faster, faster!" try your best to be methodical. Trying to come, especially with a new partner, can be a little like attempting to pick up mercury after the thermometer has broken, so the less distraction (such as a too-fast friction) as she gets close, the better.

The Main Event

Yes, I know genital penetration is supposed to be just another phase of the pleasure cycle and all that, but do I seem like somebody who cares how things are "supposed" to be when it comes to sex? Most men and women continue to regard dick in pussy as "the real thing," and I'm not just talking about former presidents, either.

After whatever reciprocal attentions your partner may devote to bringing you up to full strength, it will eventually be time to fuck. If you've both been effective at promoting each other's arousal, you'll be ready at that same time, and you'll know when that time has come. Men have been somewhat traumatized in recent years over hurrying this part, but waiting too long is no better. When she flops her legs open and fingers herself while she looks into your eyes and utters welcoming comments, I think you can assume it's time to make your grand entrance.

Of course, in this day and age, at least in the early phases of a sexual relationship, there may have to be a brief intermission for the application of a condom. This is a delicate moment that, if mishandled, can pretty much undo the best efforts of the two of you thus far. But it need not. If condoms are being used, be sure you've brought your favorite (all right, then, the least disliked) brand. Until you're comfortable with each other, and you know her skill level when it comes to lending a helping hand or mouth, it may be best to encourage her to simply provide visual stimulation while you put it on, avoiding fumbling distractions at a delicate time. And no, it won't feel the same inside her as bare tissue for either one of you. Get over it.

When it comes to intercourse, remember that the athletic positions you love to watch in porn videos are unlikely to feel very good at home. We do these positions for the benefit of the camera, but they're not often practical in the real world. You'd be surprised at how many calf cramps and backaches performers endure during a long scene. We're pros, and we can deal with what the job requires, much like athletes and dancers. However, most women I've been with enjoy fairly standard variations on face-to-face and rear-entry configurations, and, off camera, I'm no different. The more extreme positions from the *Kama Sutra* may be good fun for a minute or so at best, but you shouldn't, and won't, be expected to try out for Cirque du Soleil every time you make love. Instead, go with what feels good to the two of you, and you'll be fine. Some momentary inspiration that seemed a good idea at the time might be impossible to sustain, so don't be stubborn.

Starting with the much-maligned but still perfectly lovely "mis-

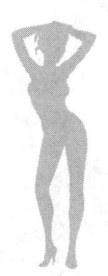

sionary" position, kneel between her legs and press your cock firmly against her pussy. If she's ready, you'll sink easily into her, and she'll grab your butt. Slide all the way in and rest your full weight on her for several breaths, as you hold her, make eye contact, kiss her, and slowly grind your hips. Women's hips are designed for load bearing as well as childbearing, so, unless you're a sumo wrestler, your mass settling in on top of her will be a glorious moment of surrender to pleasure. This completes the circuit, stimulates her clit, and encourages that distinctly feminine delight in feeling utterly pinned and deeply penetrated.

Again, it doesn't matter whether this pleasure is bred in the bone or instilled by social conditioning, most especially not when you're experiencing it. The censorious presence of feminist theorists telling you that missionary-position sex is patriarchal and oppressive is no more constructive in the bedroom than that of puritanical clerics telling you that anything else is lewd and improper. Just settle in and enjoy it.

When your partner starts to grind against you, stroking her insides with your cock, make sure to push and tuck your hips all the way forward on the in-stroke to complete the motion. If you don't follow through, you'll feel mechanical and robotic, which sucks. For variation, you can "climb" up on her a bit, forcing the top edge of your cock over her clit and vestibule with each penetration as it also presses your glans into her deeper recesses. If you drop down with your weight, the muscles at the entrance to her pussy will act as a fulcrum, angling your cock more toward her G-spot while nicely stretching her vaginal opening as your pubic mound rubs her clit. You'll find your best rhythm by experimentation. Try slowing down and speeding up, sliding straight in and out, and swiveling your hips. The trick is to keep a constant backbeat without slipping into monotonous hammering, the dreaded, unrelenting, cervix-thumping jackhammer motion that porn pros call "rabbit fucking." If you're much past the age of consent, there's no excuse for this all-too-common bad habit.

Get up onto your hands and knees, and her fingers can reach her clit. You'll also enjoy more freedom of movement in your hips to get a good pounding going. Putting her knees over your elbows intensifies this effect. Putting her knees over your shoulders does so even more. This is among the most deeply penetrating of positions, so if you're a well-endowed guy, beware of painful bottoming out. Lowering your weight carefully, your cock will stretch her already splayed pussy even farther, increasing the sensation of girth—generally a good thing. You'll also be aiming directly at her G-spot as you slide in—never a bad thing. Alternate wind sprints of hard pounding with slower, more sensual movements. As you lie completely on her body, kiss while you fuck, until it seems time to change positions. If you're fortunate, she'll be orgasmic from the combination of fucking and grinding and will be able to orgasm with you inside of her. Having a woman writhing and bucking on your cock while she comes is the kind of moment you tend to remember long after. It may be as much a tribute to her orgasmic capacity as to your lovemaking technique, but either way it's never wrong to take it as a compliment.

Likewise, if it doesn't happen, she may be a woman who comes primarily from external stimulation, and neither of you should regard her lack of orgasmic response to penetration as a failure on either person's part. When I deal in detail with the many varieties of orgasmic experience a bit later, you'll see that every woman comes in a different way, and often the same woman comes in different ways, depending on the circumstances. Loading the process with value judgments does nothing good for either of you.

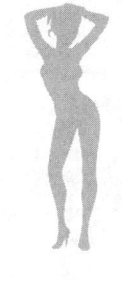

Rear-entry positions are probably the most popular for both men and women, though not all are willing to admit it. The anatomical fit is almost ideal, but there are emotional concerns regarding intimacy and modesty that sometimes inhibit the full enjoyment of this most animalistic form of coupling. I do not, therefore, recommend simply flipping your partner over and impaling her without warning. A gentlemanly suggestion, at least in the early phases of a relationship, is likely to garner a more favorable response.

There are several variations on the basic "doggy style," all of them good. There's something so primal about being taken from behind that it's hard not to be swept up in the energy of it. Then there are the practical advantages: A woman can be a bit more active when not pinned underneath you, and she gets an added jolt when your balls slap against her clit. She can also masturbate while fucking in this position without getting in your way (though if her nails are too long, you'll feel them brushing against your balls on the in-stroke, which may be distracting). With some practice, she can wield a vibrator from underneath, intensifying the internal sensations. Press her butt cheeks apart with your hands (remember, big muscle groups like deep stimulation) and ease yourself inside as far as you can comfortably go. She should make happy noises. Start rocking slowly, using her hips to pull her to you, and build up your momentum. One drawback to rear-entry positions is a tendency to lose communication with your partner. Don't be afraid to solicit some input regarding speed and stroke. It's no fun for her when you start jamming away while she's still in first gear, and not much for you if she goes stiff and rigid just as you're getting into the swing.

A favorite variation is to place a small, firm pillow under her hips and then collapse her onto it while you're still connected, your legs on the outside of hers. If you're on the long side, her butt will take up those couple of extra inches, and you'll be less likely to plunge too deeply. If you kneel back, it will change the angle of your cock and provide an amazing visual of her prone body and your penetrating penis. Pressing your hands firmly into her butt cheeks and spreading them apart will, as we say in porn, open her to camera as well as feel really good to both of you.

If it's been discussed, a gloved, lubed-up thumb or finger in her butt can send her soaring but if done without prior consent is also likely to send you flying. We'll deal with the specifics of anal stimulation during vaginal intercourse in greater detail in our chapter on anal sex, but in keeping with my general view that anal play needn't be divorced from other forms of lovemaking, I like to plant the idea wherever it seems relevant.

If you crawl up her body a bit, your cock will be positioned toward her G-spot, the benefits of which will become instantly apparent. Alternate grinding with pumping, noting which stroke she prefers. If you're very much heavier than she is, hold your weight up on your forearms to avoid that unpleasant suffocating-in-the-mattress sensation. If she's strong, lie still and let her fuck you back by clenching and relaxing her butt muscles. In this position, judicious hair pulling and neck or shoulder biting adds a pleasant frisson or two. For best results, time these actions to coincide with your deepest thrusts, then let go and pull back at the same moment. It's a highly swoon-inducing combination of delights.

If you feel or know that your cock is thinner than she'd prefer, or if you need more friction than is possible from just her muscle contractions, invest in a "realistic" cyberskin dildo. These toys are a little softer and feel more fleshlike than regular dildos. Get one with balls attached (they make a handy-dandy handle), put a condom on it, including over

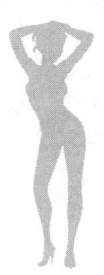

the balls (they're hard to keep clean otherwise), and slide it in beside your cock, balls up. You can pull it out as you withdraw and push it in when you return, or you can just keep it still and fuck next to it. Either way, she'll feel tighter to you and more thoroughly stuffed from within. You can always use technology to supplement your natural gifts.

If there's one consistency in porn, it's that the cocks on display are, almost to a one, 2 to 7 inches longer than the national average of 5.5 inches. It's to be expected, as the larger variety are more, well, theatrical than the regular kind and lend themselves better to the particular demands of the job: to fuck deeply and still be able to pull out enough for the camera to see the action. Such cocks serve as fantasy totems and are perfect for the dreamworld of screen sex: More! Bigger! Bouncier! Harder! I can handle most any guy once, but to really get to the wild abandon I'm seeking, he has to be of a size where my knees can be over his shoulders, as I love it that way. How you make love to us is far more important than your having a big dick. Being hung like a horse will get you lots of looky-loos but few repeat offers. We just like to be able to say "I had a guy this big once and lived to tell the tale." Women who really, truly, need a much-bigger-than-average guy, often called "size queens," are as rare as the men they seek. May they find each other. In all my days of having sex, I've only met a dozen or so. Most of us are much happier with more conventional equipment.

What if you're shorter than the national average, or thinner? Using your understanding of anatomy and physics, you can do a lot to create the illusion of girth or length. Whatever you do, avoid any surgery that promises a change in penis size or shape. Such "fixes" are expensive, painful, and don't work. Better to put that energy into coming to terms with what you've got to work with and the money toward a great vacation. Just as you find it annoying to be with a woman who constantly obsesses about a particular body part, so, too, do we dislike being with a man who bedevils himself and us with his anatomical insecurities. Besides, men who are "average" or less are better suited to anal sex, no minor advantage to be sure.

When my partner is extra well padded, I've often enjoyed "scissors" with him, as he's lovely to lazily rub my clit against. Instead of your legs being on the inside or outside of hers, they are intertwined: yours-hers-yours-hers. Your cock may not penetrate as deeply, but, again, it doesn't need to if her introitus and clit are being amply stimulated. You won't miss the deeper penetration either, as your cock will be stroked along its entirety. In addition, she can do a lot of the work, "using" you to masturbate.

"Cowgirl," or feminine superior, is a great position and often the only one from which a woman can climax during intercourse. I prefer it when my partner is propped up in bed or in a chair as opposed to flat on his back. I straddle his hips and slide him inside. With him sitting up, it's easy to kiss, and I'm not holding myself up. My hips have more freedom to move, and the combination of his swirling cock and my clit grinding away on his lower abdomen is yummy. If he has a bit of a tummy, even better! If you like, she can balance on her feet, with her arms around your neck, and bounce up and down while you cradle her butt cheeks. It's a workout but worth it! If she wants you flat on your back, let her have it that way, instead. Remember that in this position you also have excellent access to breasts, nipples, lips, and other not-to-be-neglected erogenous zones.

Then there is the favorite of porn directors, "reverse cowgirl," in which she sits on your cock while facing your feet. You can be propped up or lying flat. Keep your butt and legs firmly tensed, the better for her to bounce on you. You can spread her cheeks apart, spank them, or,

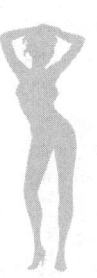

if this has already been mutually agreed upon, put a gloved, lubed thumb in her butt. The view is fantastic, especially if you have a mirror next to the bed, which is why this position plays so well on camera. It can also be uncomfortable after a fairly short time, bending your dick too far forward and stressing her calf muscles, so it's best as a short interlude between more practical positions. She can also assume this position as you sit in a chair, which is a real quad burner.

I love "spooning." Nothing is nicer than rubbing your butt up against a guy, only to be greeted by a woody. A little lube and *bang!* You're in. It's a bit more difficult to get traction in this position, but it's a lovely, lazy way to stay connected. She has to work a bit harder to fuck you back, but it's still nice because neither of you has to hold anything back. It's a great way to wake up someone who likes morning sex (or middle-of-the-night sex). From here, it's easy to caress her hair, neck, and breasts, though a proper buildup to orgasm may prove daunting.

Another porn favorite that can be good for home use is the "pile driver." This is a very rambunctious, athletic position that can be a lot of fun if your partner is limber and your legs are strong. I've seen it develop from a cowgirl-on-the-couch that slips to the floor as well as from starting with her rolling onto her shoulders with her knees near her head, and him dipping his cock into her from above. You're then able to fuck her by bending your knees and doing short squats, very fast. *Whew!* You can get more depth and traction if you straddle her, one foot near her butt and one near one shoulder in the front, assuming a lunge position (one leg straight and one bent). A straight cock works better than a curved one for this configuration, and, once again, it's more likely to be an occasional variant than a regular fave.

Sooner or later, it'll be time for you to come, whether or not she's had an orgasm yet. I know many books say not to even begin intercourse unless she's come once or twice, but if I used that yardstick, I'd never get any (and neither would my lover)! When you're done and cleaned up a bit (baby wipes to the rescue!), hold her close and ask if there's anything she needs or if there's something you can do for her. If she needs more, she'll request that you help her come, either for the umpteenth time or the first. Hold and caress her while she uses a vibrator on her clit, or use your magic fingers inside of her while she buzzes or diddles herself to ecstasy. If you've chosen the right partner, she'll welcome your offer of help and be happy to tell you what she needs from you.

When she's done with her orgasm(s), cuddling is almost always welcome, though I do know a few women who don't much care for it, even after sex. This is the time when emotions are close to the surface and our hearts have been softened from exertion and pleasure. If she, or you, uses the "L" word, don't freak. You're experiencing love at that very moment, and it doesn't necessarily mean that it will continue when the afterglow has faded. The love you may feel is real and true and possibly transitory. Loving behavior elicits loving feelings, which is how it should be. Don't cling to it or make it into something more than it is. If it's the beginning of True Love, that will become apparent over time. I love all of my lovers while we're playing, which adds a lot to our pleasure, but I don't confuse it with the love I feel for my life partner.

A word about her orgasm: You can help her out a lot, but you can't "give" her one, and she shouldn't expect you to. You can only make it safe or fun for her to have it on her own. I've been with women who come with alarming and exciting frequency and ease from oral sex, fingers, toys, and dicks, even from humping a leg. Hell, I knew one woman who could come when she wore tight jeans! Then there are women like me, who come once, hard, but it's not easy to get there, sorta like guys. Still

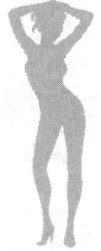

others reach their first orgasm of the night easily, with subsequent ones taking more and more effort (gotta love those vibrators!), while still others have a hard time getting to the first one, but all the rest follow easily once the threshold has been breached. Forget what you see in porn; those are performances. Don't let your masculine ego trap you into feeling angry, annoyed, or inadequate because your partner needs mechanical help to come, since all technology does is save you effort. You're a guy, so get into the groove of using cool gizmos to help her get there. I mean, what's hotter than watching a woman bring herself off while you offer boob support? We'll explore the deeper mysteries of the orgasmic response in due course. Meantime, give yourself and your partner a break.

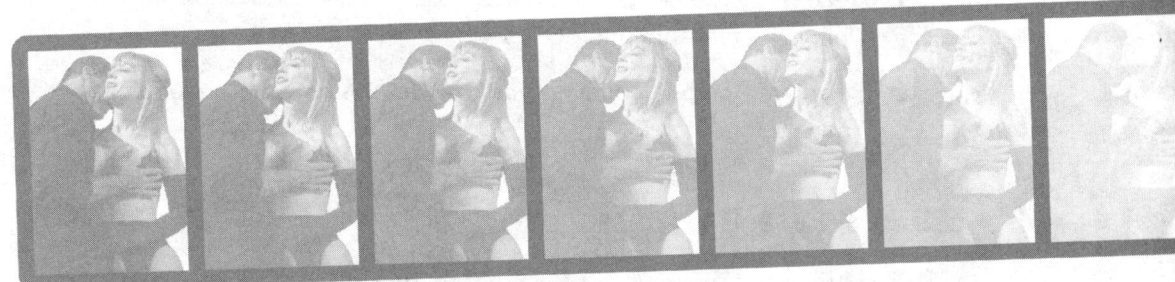

WOMAN-HANDLING WINNERS

1 · *Know how our bodies work so we can relax under your touch.*

2 · *You know that joke about how men won't call when they say they will and come when they say they won't? Make sure we're not talking about you.*

3 • *Our bodies aren't fragile; our feelings can be.* Handle the former with confidence and the latter with caution.

4 • *We know you like to look, and that's fine.* Just remember to look into our eyes once in a while.

5 • *Slow down.* Even slower than that would be good.

6 • *Once you find something that works, stick with it.* We'll let you know if we're ready to move on.

7 • *Remember that you're making love to our whole bodies,* not just the critical few square inches.

8 • *Change it up.* Unless we're in a preorgasmic groove and don't want it short-circuited, feel free to initiate a switch of position or approach. Creativity is a rare virtue in a lover.

9 • *And let us do the same.* We like to get creative, too, especially when we feel safe and accepted.

10 • *If you're going to come outside, ask first where we'd prefer the payload.*

DON'T EVEN GO THERE

1 • *No acting out anything from a porn tape without prior negotiation.* We don't want to feel you're more into a two-dimensional woman than a live one.

2 • *No snide comments on our bodies.* If you don't find us attractive, don't invite us to your bed.

3 • *We hate 'em, too, but no bitching or whining about condoms.* It's just how it is.

4 • *Careful with the "L" word.* You may say it in the heat of passion, but it will echo in our heads all night.

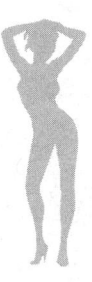

5 • *Whatever you're asking for, no means no, and once should be enough.* It doesn't mean ask us again five minutes later to see if we've changed our minds. If we do, you'll be the first to know.

6 • *No medals will be awarded for the number of orgasms facilitated.* That's pressure we don't need.

7 • *Easy on the clit.* You'll have better luck in the surrounding neighborhood than working away at the most sensitive spot.

8 • *Careful with that dick, Eugene.* When you're pounding away toward the finish line, the difference between *ooh* and *ouch* is about a centimeter shy of the cervix.

9 • *Don't be afraid to let us know you're having a good time.* However deep into your thing you may be at the moment, come around to pay an occasional compliment. We have our insecurities too.

10 • *Don't forget to shave.* Razor burn on the puss is a major drag, and that stubble thing is so ten minutes ago.

Chapter 9

MAKING LOVE TO MEN: INSERTING TAB A IN SLOT B

love men. I love how unlike women they are when turned on and how like women they can be when turned on. I love their willingness to let a woman take the lead or to take the lead themselves. I love how directly sex speaks to and from the hearts of men, compelling me to speak directly also. It was my enduring fascination with male sexuality that propelled my initial career choices. More than twenty years on, I still learn something new about men every time I'm sexual with one. My most important discovery (and I keep coming back to it) is that there's less difference between genders and more diversity among individuals when it comes to sex and what we each want from it than contemporary gender politics would have us believe. I've learned that men are as complex, sexually and emotion-

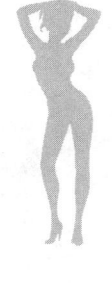

ally, as women, though in different areas and for different reasons. I've learned that there's no "understanding men" but only understanding a particular man. While this chapter is addressed primarily to my female readers, smart guys will be wise to give it as much attention as they will the information specifically intended to enhance their knowledge of women's preferences. When it comes to sex, there really is no such thing as too much information.

There are basically three ways for you to have intercourse with a man. You can be still, letting him penetrate you as he wishes, allowing his heat to fill you while you do nothing more than squeeze your pelvic muscles on the out-stroke and relax on the in-stroke. You can fuck each other equally, adjusting your rhythms until you achieve a satisfying synchronous motion. As a third alternative, you can have him remain still inside of you with his weight behind his dick as you wiggle, thrust, and grind against him to achieve the perfect friction. Getting your hip joints to loosen up may take a bit of practice, but, as with dancing, you'll feel less clumsy with repetition. The two of you can cycle through these changes at will, lingering on any variation from seconds to minutes for as long as the sensation remains pleasurable. If your motions get a little disjointed, be still and let him find his groove. Why? Understanding that he's the one who needs to maintain an erection, err on the side of letting him do what he needs to keep his edge. If you're performing with the kind of relaxed attention that is as effective in sex as it is mountain climbing, you'll know when he's got his groove back and it's safe to start improvising again. He receives pleasure from you "taking" yours, so don't hesitate to steer the situation to where you'd like it to go.

One of the easiest ways for him to experience the satisfaction of receptivity, besides the hand/blow job, is for you to get on top. The view is great (boobs in the face!), and he doesn't have to worry about fucking you "wrong." This is also one of the easiest positions in which you can come through intercourse, since you can adjust the angle, depth, and speed of penetration and give yourself and your partner easy clitoral access. For me, this works best when my partner is propped at about a forty-five-degree incline and I straddle his hips. The grinding and stroking I do rubs my clit the right way (if he's not too skinny) while his cock operates like a swizzle stick inside of me, hitting all my great spots. I can also lean back on my arms and slide around, giving him an eye— or hand—full of the goods.

While I'm not a fan of "cowgirl" with my partner flat on his back, it does provide a great visual for both partners. You'll make a memorable impression if you sit on his cock and then get up onto your toes, resting your knees against your arms for support and leverage. Now, simply bounce up and down on him. It may not be the most orgasmic configuration for you, but it's super-hot to see his dick disappear into you so effortlessly. You can vary the routine by leaning forward, offering your tits or bringing your face close for deep, intimate kissing. If you're feeling the need for emotional connection on a particular occasion, this can be an ideal way to make contact.

A good feminine-superior variation is to kneel over him while facing his feet, which works well even when he's flat on his back. This will tilt his dick down into your G-spot while you rock back and forth. He gets an amazing view of your backside and can slip a thumb into your butt for some really hot sensations, if that's on the menu (more to come in the chapter on anal pleasure). It's easy to spank from here, too, another special treat we'll explore at length later. In this position you can also use a vibrator on your clit fairly easily. Some men find the buzzing

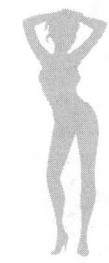

sensation irritating, which is to be respected, or the vibrator itself somehow competitive, which is to be dispelled by your reassuring attention to the part he plays in your heightened enjoyment. You may feel awkward about "using" him for your sexual pleasure, but in my experience, men like to feel useful, especially when it comes to sex, and don't feel much guilt at using you in a similar fashion. Take a page from the guys' handbook and let go of your guilt about simply having a good time.

After you've really revved up his motor, you'll probably both be ready for some solid "missionary" fucking. This position has taken a lot of heat over the years, both from feminist ideologues and swing-from-the-chandelier liberationists, but it's a perennial favorite for many good reasons: kissing, hugging, eye contact, clit rubbing, and, to be totally un-PC about it, lying back and taking it like a woman (after you've inspired him to give it like a man). I always have a firm, small pillow (a buckwheat-hull–filled cushion is ideal) on the bed to put under my hips, facilitating maximum penetration where my vaginal canal is most accommodating.

Once he's inside, I love to have him lower his entire weight onto me, sliding his cock deep into my *posterior fornix* (don't forget those spots—quiz to follow!) as we press our bodies together and breathe deeply. This lets us relax into the rhythm of fucking, a delicious transition from the preliminaries to the main event. He can make little hip thrusts, and I can squeeze my pelvic muscles in return. After a few breaths, we'll start to grind our hips. When mine are thrust forward fully, he can't help but penetrate me more deeply as my clit is pressed and rubbed between our pubic bones. Moving our hips in unison, we relax into a timeless, synchronous motion. I like to squeeze him intermittently with my thighs, pushing him off me for brief intervals, then relaxing suddenly, letting him land on me that much harder. It's a challenging workout and a great way to be active while lying on my back.

If you reach under his arms and pull him toward you as you thrust upward with your pelvis while squeezing him with your thighs, you'll generate even more dynamic tension. I like to get myself panting and raise my pulse like this, because it makes it all the more fun to then go "floppy" and be totally receptive. If he thinks you're actually trying to push him off you, reassure him that you're not, and he'll continue with renewed vigor.

With your knees up, wrap your arms around his neck and then bend your elbows, bringing your forearms back to your head so that your upper arms are resting on his shoulders. Push down with your arms (great triceps and lat workout) as you pull up with your legs (good for the lower abs too) and hold on for as long as you can while you continue to fuck each other vigorously. In about half a minute or so, with your heart racing, exhale as you relax completely. It's a great, swoony rush, and you'll be rewarded with an extra burst of passion from him. It's a kind of struggle, but without the fear and danger of the real thing. You're not going for the gold here, so a few moves of this type, interspersed with less challenging strokes, raise the temperature a few notches without overheating either one of you.

People have long asked me how I've gotten my abs in such good shape. I tell them it's easy: Regularly making love to a person who outweighs me by fifty to eighty pounds is a great workout! For example, while in missionary, I'll hold up my head as I watch his cock disappear inside me. Before I know it, I've completed a painless twenty-minute upper-ab crunch. If he rests his weight completely on me, it's a great lower-ab workout for me to use my hips to move his weight around. The

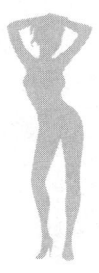

secondary health benefits of vigorous lovemaking may not figure prominently in your motivations, but they are among the many rewards of an active and well-rounded sex life.

I have exactly zero statistical evidence for this opinion, but my own experience and anecdotal testimony suggest that rear-entry positions are solid favorites among experienced lovers. This is partially a by-product of our sexual anatomy and in no small measure a barometer of our comfort level with the more animalistic aspects of intercourse. They don't call it "doggy style" for nothing. With the exception of whales and primates, coitus is pretty much a front-to-back engagement for all mammals.

At the above-the-neck level, where so much of the sexual experience takes place, rear-entry positions can facilitate fantasy, since, without face-to-face contact, you can each be whomever you want. This "impersonality" can be troubling to some, but on a purely selfish level, doggy style is a perennial favorite, in part, for that very reason. I have to admit that I'm always a bit suspicious of those who find rear-entry intercourse distasteful for its "lack of intimacy." There is an intimacy in allowing myself to be both my lover's unique partner and an imaginary stranger at the same time and letting myself visit those hidden places in my erotic imagination, too, that is every bit as real and close as looking deeply into each other's eyes during the act.

We lucky humans are particularly adapted to appreciate penetration from behind, both as givers and receivers. Your partner is able to enjoy the visual splendor of your butt, which is a universal sexual totem for men as well as a wonderfully pornographic view of his cock sliding in and out of you. You get to experience the purist sensation of penetration, free of the necessity of supporting his body weight or yours. In this utterly primal position, you can both really let go. His hips can loosen up more easily with his knees as a fulcrum, and you can swing yours, with your elbows providing a sturdy pivot point. It's a lovely, lazy girl's way to get boned, and you can easily reach your clit while the two of you try out various rhythms.

Here again, if anal play is part of the deal, he can easily slip a gloved, lubed finger or thumb into your ass, either as an added sensation heightener or a prelude to more serious anal stimulation. Try arching your back to vary the points of internal contact (and to present yourself even more alluringly) or putting your chest on the bed, which lifts your backside higher. If the resulting penetration is too deep, have him do what porn dudes do and "cheat" the angle of his thrusts. A guy often needs to "hit bottom" at the end of the stroke, but if your pussy is too shallow in this position (as it often can be), have him "open up" a bit and slam his hip into your butt cheek instead of hammering his cock into your cervix. You'll both have the benefit of hard banging without the uncomfortable side effects. You can also experiment with bringing your knees closer together or spreading them farther apart, thus raising or lowering the point of connection for the most favorable geometry.

I also like "collapsed doggy," with me on my stomach, a firm pillow under my hips, my legs straight behind me, his legs outside of mine. Since my butt is big, a "too long" guy can fit better because of the additional padding. He can sit back on his heels for a long perspective or climb up on me, which also directs his cock to my G-spot and takes up a few of those extra inches. This way, he can fuck more freely without either of us worrying about that errant poke. As a great butt workout, have him stay still while you "fuck" him, simply by squeezing and relaxing your cheeks. Try it; you'll see!

Standing rear-entry positions are a fun challenge, requiring a bit of attention to balance but allowing for a great variety of sensations sim-

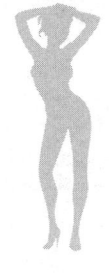

ply by adjusting your stance. Fully bend over, holding your ankles if you're agile enough. Try pulling yourself up straight until you're nearly standing back to chest. You can try this position with knees together or apart, straight or bent; in high heels; flat-footed; or barefoot on tiptoe. If he grabs your hips to hold you close, grind and wiggle against him while he enjoys the spectacle and you share the stimulation.

"Lap dancing" is a personal favorite, especially when the dick in question is sized and shaped so you can rest your full weight in your partner's lap without discomfort. If you do it in front of a mirror, you can see for yourself how sexy you are. The chair should be narrow enough so you can easily hold on to the arms but big enough to allow both you and your partner freedom of movement. Have him sit in the chair and jerk his penis for you as you do a few moments of a sexy dance. Turn to show him your bottom and let him pet, squeeze, or spank it. Have him hold his dick by the base and slowly sink onto it. You can rock back and forth, grind in circles, or stroke him by holding up your weight with your arms and rocking back and forth, using your feet as a balance point. You'll feel almost weightless, and he can easily push you back and forth as you ride him high. If you have an over-stuffed chair, it's fun to straddle him and fuck face-to-face. Being on your knees allows you more room to maneuver and a lot of leverage when you hook your feet over his thighs.

One position that combines the advantages of rear-entry and full-body contact is the so-called "spoon," in which you both stretch out on one hip and he slips into you from behind. Though your movements will be somewhat limited by the forward tilt of your vaginal canal, you'll be able to squirm together like dolphins, intertwine your limbs, keep your faces in close contact, and use your bodies as leverage against each other. As your movements speed up toward a climax, your bodies will naturally separate in order to deepen the penetration, but the sensation of being held by the shoulders and pulled back onto a rigid cock is satisfying in a thoroughly primal fashion.

A variant of this approach, called "scissors" in porn, has you on your back with your partner on top of you, your legs intertwined. This is best for sexy, orgasmic grinding and wiggling more than for thrusting but feels very good with a well-padded boyfriend. A vertical approach to this position, in which the woman props herself up on her shoulders, throws her legs back over her head, and presents herself bottom up so the man can squat and enter her from above is called a "pile driver." As the name suggests, it allows for deep and powerful thrusting, but I only recommend it for the strong and limber, more as a fun interlude for a few moments than a standard part of a regular repertoire. When you see us do it in the movies, remember that we are trained professionals, and while you can try many of the things we do at home safely enough, you may find they look better than they feel.

For all the variations to be found in the *Kama Sutra,* most couples discover two or three types of connections that always work and to which they always return, sooner or later. I'm no different. My home positions are fairly typical variations of rear entry and face-to-face. This isn't boring; it's what functions best for us and for the way our bodies fit together. Your favorites will undoubtedly be somewhat different. I tried a new position with a new lover not long ago and it was fantastic, but nothing I'd be able to re-create at home, since its success was predicated on both his body type (tall and slender) and his dick type (long and thin). There is no optimal configuration for intercourse beyond that which suits the two of you at the moment. Sex is not a competitive sport, and there are no extra points to be had for working your way through record numbers of positions in the shortest possible time.

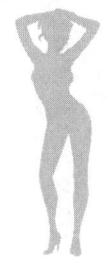

Variety may be the spice of life, but consistency and reliability are its bedrock. Again, modern pornography offers us both useful and contradictory examples in this regard. Porn performers are sexual athletes for whom physically demanding couplings in less-than-comfortable circumstances are all in a day's work. Sex for you isn't and shouldn't be hard labor or triathlon training. It's fun and exciting to try new things, but the comfort and confidence with which you play the old standards are rich elements of long-term relationships whose benefits should not be underestimated. Steering the proper course between monotony and perpetual performance anxiety is a key element in the art of maintaining sexual heat over a protracted period of time.

Taking Matters in Hand

Now that we've covered the basics of intercourse that apply in most situations, what happens when we encounter the unexpected? The Declaration of Independence may declare that all men are created equal, but that hasn't been my experience. I've known a lot of dicks in my time: big ones and small ones, thin ones and thick ones, short ones and long ones, straight ones and curved or bent ones, in every possible configuration. I did the math, and it's well into the miles of dick that I've had, and not all of them were a perfect fit. How do I manage all these variables (Hint: It's a lot easier when you have to work with a guy only once) and, more important, how do you? By being practical minded and unafraid of honesty, you can achieve a workable accommodation. If anyone's always worrying about hurting or being hurt, there can be no letting go or surrender, and the attempt will always be a chore, or worse.

There are guys who tell me, "I've got ten inches and can go all night," to which I always reply, "Cut off four inches and call me in the morning." I don't know about you, but there's a definite limit to what I can or want to take inside me, no matter how aroused I am. I call such supersized men "special-occasion cocks," as it's an effort for me to make love with such guys. Part of the fun of sex is working up to the point where it's "balls to the wall": fucking hard with total abandon and sheer animal passion. If I have to keep part of my logical brain switched on to prevent an ovary from being dislodged or if he has to hold back for fear of uncomfortably banging my viscera, no one has the good time for which I engage in recreational sex, and we should switch to a blow job and have done with it.

If a guy is too long to comfortably fuck me in a more conventional manner, I'll try a variation on missionary. With my legs open, I'll have him start penetration. I'll bring my legs in slowly, until my ankles are crossed and his legs are outside of mine. If he climbs up toward me a little bit, his cock is forced down, sliding over my clit in a delicious fashion. Even better, with my cervix safely out of the line of fire, he can then fuck me as hard as he wishes. I can grab his butt and urge him to let his passion out.

If penetration simply isn't an option, I'll still lie on my back with my ankles crossed, but I'll take his cock in my lubed-up fists so he can fuck my hands. His balls or my knuckles will rub on my clit, and we can kiss while he really goes for it. This is also a great way to "fuck" safely if there are no condoms available. If I lie on my stomach with a firm pillow under my hips and he straddles me, he can fuck the space between my legs, sliding his cock over my clit. If we're standing up, I'll lube up my inner thighs, cross my ankles, and have him, from behind, fuck the space between my vulva and legs. His cock will naturally ride over my clit, ending up in my lubed-up fist. These "unconventional" ap-

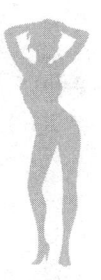

proaches let him cut loose without putting either of us in uncomfortable situations.

Another fun alternative for those whose partner has an extra-long unit is to sit astride him, lube up his shaft as it lies on his abdomen, and hump it. If he's truly long enough, his glans will never touch your vulva (yes, I've seen plenty of cocks that were that long!), so you can grease up your hand and play with his glans as you rub yourself to ecstasy.

Men endowed with too much girth for a particular pussy represent a different challenge. When a guy is too thick, I've found that lubing up my thighs and having him fuck the space in between, either from the front or back, is about as much as I can do, besides giving him a hand job or blow job. Starting on top can help, since I can ease him inside, but if that takes too long he's likely to deflate, which sorta sucks. Face-to-face can also work, with him feeding it in slowly, but you'll still find yourself holding back if he's uncomfortably stretching your insides. While the vaginal canal is highly pliable and ultimately designed to give birth, no woman would choose this as a nightly experience. These guys need to find those women for whom there is no such thing as too much meat.

A bend or curve in a man's erection may dictate certain compromises as well, depending on its severity. If his erection winds left, start in missionary, pull your legs up and together, and roll over onto your right hip, thereby aiming the end of his cock at your G-spot. From there, you can play with your clit, and he can fuck normally without hurting your ovaries. If his erection curves or bends right, you'll want to roll over onto your left hip, again so he'll hit the optimal spot. The more extreme his swerve, the fewer comfortable options you have. If he curves up, rather than to one side, you can forget the sitting-on-him-facing-his-ankles approach, but he'll be great at missionary or doggy.

If he has a downward tilt, knees-over-the-shoulder missionary is great, guiding the missile perfectly into your posterior fornix for a delicious, cervix-sparing sensation. From the rear, it should rub perfectly over your G-spot. One of my best one-night stands ever was like this, and I still think about him over a decade later!

When it comes to anatomical incompatibilities, there's usually plenty of will and therefore almost always a way. However, in contemplating long-term sexual relationships, the commitment to finding that way every single time you have sex may eventually sap the necessary motivation and lead to excessive late-night TV viewing. I'm up for trying to fit square pegs into round holes on an occasional basis, but I wouldn't consider any man whose cock didn't feel good inside me under most circumstances as potential mate material. If you find that you really don't like that part of him, eventually you'll be likely to tire of the rest as well.

Ups and Downs

During the course of a lovemaking session, especially when a couple is new together, a man may lose and regain his erection several times. This is normal! In porn, all the footage of the guy struggling to get or keep his dick hard is edited out, doubtless adding to the already daunting performance anxiety a man must overcome to function. When a woman may lubricate and dry out several times during a romp, the effect is subtle, invisible, and readily overcome with a bit of lube. A man's emotional state is clear for all to see, which makes him vulnerable emotionally as well as physically. In a society that defines masculinity in very narrow terms, men are inclined to view their erections,

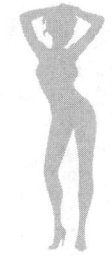

or lack thereof, as the measure of their worth. Unfortunately, biology often proves uncooperative in intimate circumstances, and it does no good to blame him or yourself for the unpredictability of a hard-on. If even a moment's thought about work, money, kids, etc., enters his mind, or if the phone rings or the cat starts scratching at the bedroom door, spontaneous detumescence may occur without warning.

If, or more likely when, this happens, your response will do much to determine what follows. Your feelings of frustration, inadequacy, and/ or disappointment will almost certainly be less intense than his (it's his anatomy that's the source of the problem, after all), and your ability to offer reassurance is the best hope for a desired resurrection. Reconnect on the mental and emotional levels before focusing your attention on his dick. A sudden crash dive may only increase his performance anxiety, and failure to inspire it may only add your insecurities to his. When a man loses his erection with me (as they do more than you think, and I'm supposed to be a sex goddess!), I suggest fun alternatives: cunnilingus, toys, clit play, kissing, mutual masturbation, etc. Slow, deep massage of his cock can work wonders. Be methodical and scientific about it as you manipulate his penis all the way back to the bulb. Note what makes his pelvic muscles contract, and start a tactile dialogue with them. Generally, slower and deeper stimulation is better than frantic jerking, at least until the erectile response returns. Nibble his ear lobe until he shivers. Say a few dirty things in his ear that you know he'd like. Sometimes he'll have to lend a hand of his own, so enjoy that show and add to it yourself, taking advantage of his natural response to visual stimulation (told you it would come in handy!). By relieving him of the pressure to perform, you'll enhance his ability to do just that, which will get you more of what you want. Sometimes his erection won't return, for whatever reason, and that has to be okay, too. Nonerectile ejaculations are not uncommon and shouldn't be regarded as some second-class version of "the genuine article."

There are drugs on the market to help men who have difficulty achieving or maintaining erections. It is a fact that many otherwise-healthy men are now using these drugs for recreational purposes. For reasons about which I have my suspicions, many women seem resentful of these pharmacological performance enhancers, and to them I say, "Get over it, girls." This isn't the Olympics, and reliance on chemical supports is no reflection on his intrinsic merits as a lover or on yours. If a guy's personal physician sees no harm in prescribing them, I have no problem with their use, any more than I would consider it reasonable for a man to feel threatened by my employment of my vibrator. Sometimes, the extra confidence a pill can bestow is all that's needed, even if the pill acts more or less as a placebo.

However, know that pharmaceuticals can't help a guy if his heart isn't in it and are virtually useless for men who are hoping to push past their shyness and get it on in a group situation or under other circumstances in which a natural response would be unlikely. These drugs don't inspire the libido; they merely enhance physiological processes already in operation. Pharmacologically supported or not, his erection is a response to you, not to his doctor. If your partner does use meds, don't let his erection lead the show or make you feel as if you're not appreciated or needed for his arousal. Let them give him the reassurance that his hard-on will be there when you both want it, so that you can both focus more on the feelings and emotions between the two of you. You may want to feel the pride in "doing it all" for him, but he may want to be worry free, able to pay attention to things other than his fear that he might not get it up. Let him know when it's time to "drop the dime," and use that intervening hour to sink into the mood, start the foreplay, and otherwise prepare for a rockin' good time.

In the early stages of a sexual relationship, barrier protection needs to be used until both parties have been tested for STDs. Most women and men I know don't like barriers but see them as necessary, potentially life-saving annoyances. While I suspect there may have been some understandable overreaction to the emergence of the threat of HIV, I'm concerned that we may now be reentering a period of dangerous denial precisely because of the degree of success our society has experienced in containing the risk of infection. I'm alarmed whenever young people tell me that they've engaged in unprotected intercourse with someone they don't really know because they didn't want "to spoil the mood" by insisting on precautions. Given the potential hazards involved, a few moments of uncomfortable conversation beforehand are a much smaller price to pay than the potential alternatives. Until that trip to the clinic, condoms are where it's at, so deal with it. Do not allow yourself to be talked out of responsible behavior, either by your partner or yourself.

It's the guy's job to do his masturbatory homework to find the brand of condom that, if not exactly a favorite, annoys him the least, and always to have a supply with him. And girls, don't be afraid to lend a hand, or mouth, to help him get past that fumblesome moment of getting properly dressed for the occasion. However, despite all good intentions and best efforts, it's common, especially for the first time or two with a new lover, for a man to find sustaining an erection impossible while wearing a condom.

Though this problem is less common with younger men who came of age in the era of safer sex, it can and does happen to all kinds of men under all kinds of circumstances. When it does, I immediately cease and desist trying to fuck and substitute a blow job, hand job, or whatever keeps him hard, even if it means a noncoital date. He can always assist me in coming later by helping me to masturbate. It's not always necessary to follow the porn-standard template: he eats, she eats, they fuck, and they come. If you really need something inside you for a satisfying conclusion, that's what toys are for, and there's a whole chapter about them coming up soon.

Making love to a man isn't about his penis; it's about him. Remember this simple, unassailable truth, and you'll never disappoint either one of you. Like women, men have vastly differing orgasmic responses, needing anywhere from a couple of minutes to an hour of stimulation in order to get there. If a guy has a short trigger, there are books he can use to teach himself to last longer, and he should practice on his own time. You can help by learning to read the signs of his approaching ejaculation and employing the "squeeze-and-hold" technique recommended by most sex therapists. If your partner still comes more quickly than you need for your pleasure, he can learn to use toys on you or help you to masturbate while you wait for his next erection. He's probably already hypersensitive about his low orgasmic threshold, and shaming

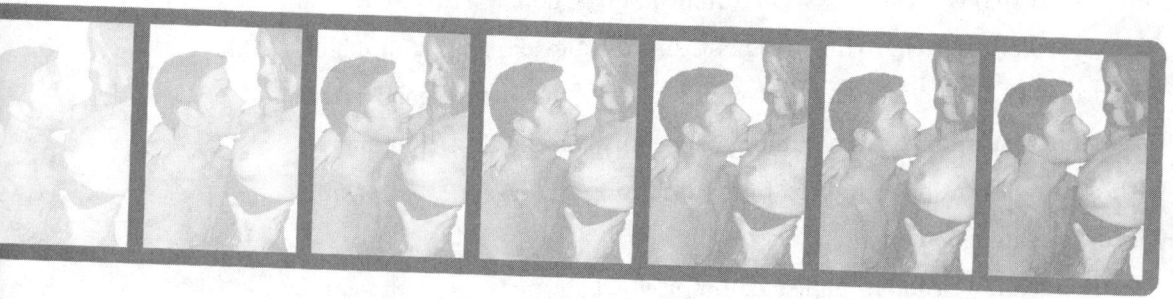

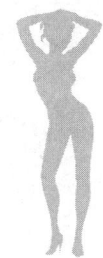

him for it is unlikely to improve matters. If he's worth your time, learn together how to extend his ability to hold off.

Other men have the opposite "problem," in that they can't come in less than thirty, or even sixty, minutes unless they're masturbating. This is not a reflection on you. Unlike a hair-trigger guy, who can train his responses to slow down, it's difficult to get a longtime lover to speed up, even if he wants to. If you're done fucking and he's not, help in other ways. Hands and mouths come to mind. If those aren't enough and you're getting tired, lie back and encourage him to jerk off on your chest. Don't shut him out, but don't exhaust or frustrate yourself in the desire to satisfy him. Ultimately, men and women are both responsible for their own orgasms. You can help each other or hinder each other in accepting this fact, but in order to enjoy fulfilling sex lives, you'll have to come to terms with it sooner or later.

PENETRATION POSITIVES

1 • *There is no such thing as too much lube.* If you're naturally juicy, a little dab will do you. Otherwise, well-oiled parts wear better longer. Don't be shy about asking for more.

2 • *Let your body do the talking.* Your movements will cue your lover more effectively than reading aloud from this or any other book.

3 • *Stick with what's working.* If it feels good to you, it probably feels good to him.

4 • *Find your groove.* Subtly vary your rhythm in each position until you hit the beat.

5 • *Stay loose.* The more you can relax the rest of your body, the more effectively you'll focus energy at the point of contact.

6 • *Lend a hand.* Keep the energy level up by touching both his body and your own during intercourse.

7 • *Change it up.* If you feel your energies starting to flag, even a slight alteration in position or tempo can get you back on track.

8 • *Don't forget to fuck back!* Worthy men want to know you're liking it too.

CIRCUIT BREAKERS

1 • *No reneging on your part of the bargain.* If he's jumped through all of your presex hoops, show up and give it all you've got, with your heart and mind open.

2 • *Don't check out.* He'll know if you're counting the ceiling tiles. Try something different if you're having trouble staying focused.

3 • *Cut the chatter.* Unless your man specifically craves dirty talk, no distracting conversation while fucking.

4 • *Avoid aerobics.* Sex is a sensual form of pleasure seeking, not an athletic event. Relentless hammering gets old quick.

5 • *Stop worrying about how you look.* Right now, you're Helen of Troy to him.

6 • *Never sacrifice your own enjoyment.* It's one thing to hold an uncomfortable position for an extra minute until he gets off, quite another to endure ongoing misery with gritted teeth. Deal with that foot cramp before it ruins the mood.

7 • *Never fake it.* Pretending to like what you don't insults your dignity and his intelligence.

8 • *Don't be afraid to ask for what you want.* Chances are he'll welcome the input.

Chapter 10

ANAL SEX:
NO PAIN, ALL GAIN

s Dr. Carol Queen says, "The anus is a very democratic orifice. Everybody has one." This fact is basic to the appeal of anal play, and what's sauce for the goose is definitely sauce for the gander. I suspect certain readers of this chapter will assume that anal sex is something a man "does" to a woman, an antiquated view that undoubtedly contributes to the resentful reluctance many women feel toward the prospect. A question I hear on the road more often than I would wish is: "How do I get my wife/girlfriend to let me have anal sex with her?" Starting from the assumptions implied by the phrasing of the inquiry, I can pretty confidently predict that nothing I suggest will be of much use.

Fortunately, a younger, more adventurous, less desperately homophobic generation of sexual adventurers, male and female, seems more willing to accept the anatomical realities of anal play with far fewer preconceptions. Both men and women are capable of enjoying satisfying, pain-free anal stimulation, and men are actually equipped with some anatomical advantages in this regard. While all butts are wired to feel exquisite pleasure, the location of the prostate gland can add significantly to men's enjoyment of butt play.

Mother Nature has endowed both genders entire pelvic regions with plentiful supplies of blood and nerves, showing particular generosity to our butts. The skin of the anus and anal canal is as densely packed with sensory receptors as are our clits or dicks. Why? The brain has a vested interest in knowing precisely what is entering or exiting the body via its portals. "Transitional areas," where the boundaries of the body are breached—mouths, nostrils, ears, genitals, and, of course, anuses—are particularly sensitive, given our natural vulnerabilities in these regions. The tissues of the external sphincter and the anal canal are particularly thin and delicate, increasing their sensitivity even more, for better or worse, depending on how they're treated. You already know this to be true. If anyone has ever gotten within an eighth of an inch of your anus, haven't you found yourself suddenly extremely alert? Part of your response is conditioned, and part is purely natural. You want and need to know what's going on back there and how you feel about it.

The commonly understood meaning of the term *anal sex* implies a specific focus on penile penetration, which is certainly a common and highly enjoyable practice but by no means the only way in which our versatile rear orifices can be put to good use. I take a broader view of anal pleasure and play, which encompasses everything from delicate,

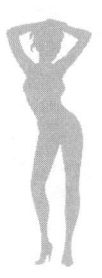

surface-only stimulation up to and including "oh-my-God-I-didn't-know-it-could-do-that" feats of relaxation and expansion. From mild to wild, it's all about finding where on the continuum of anal enjoyment you feel most comfortable. Some people take to anal play quickly and effortlessly, while others have to coax themselves along over months, or even years, a millimeter at a time. Some discover it very early in life, while others stumble onto it only after finding a particularly compatible partner. Some like and need anal play every time they have sex. For others, it's an occasional treat. And to be fair, some people never become comfortable with the idea, much less the reality, and enjoy full, rich sex lives without exploring it at all. Almost everyone desiring the delights of anal stimulation will need quite a bit of practice to settle into the intense sensations produced no other way, so a measure of adventurous determination will have much to do with the quality of the ultimate mastery of anal satisfaction.

Since anatomy and culture dictate that we spend most of our lives literally "tight assed" and since relaxation is the magic key to anal enjoyment, daring to bypass our deep conditioning about this particular body part is incredibly powerful and transformative. It's revelatory as well, since we invariably open up more than our asses in the process. Anal stimulation is an incredibly lush, voluptuous, self-centered, internal, hedonistic, and narcissistic pleasure, and claiming it, a moment at a time, reveals truths about us that can be accessed no other way. Which is not to say that learning to accept it is a simple matter. Along with the purely physical intensity of butt stimulation, we must also address the added burden of our culture's attitude toward pleasure in general, butt pleasure in particular, and what it means to like being tickled there, be it with a finger, toy, or penis.

Why (and Why Not!) Anal Sex?

While we've established that all of us have the physical equipment to enjoy anal sex in one form or another, there is still only one valid reason to pursue it: your own desire to do so. Reasons not to are equally valid and deserving of respect, which is why I devote a separate chapter to the subject and don't automatically include it in my more general descriptions of lovemaking. Though anal play is virtually always an option on my sexual menu, it is not requisite for everybody every time.

Don't do it to please another person. Don't do it if you don't want to. Don't do it if it hurts. Don't do it if you feel any pressure to do so. Butts can't lie, so don't do it to "prove" anything to anyone, including yourself. Don't do it on a dare or with someone who is drunk or high or if you are. I stress this particular point because I know that these are the conditions under which people frequently "end up" having butt sex, thereby contributing to unsatisfactory and unsafe experiences. Using drugs or alcohol to shortcut proper preparation (physical and mental) is asking for later repercussions, ranging from disappointing to uncomfortable to life threatening. If your partner is gung ho and you're reticent, find a middle ground you can both live with or give it up. Preferences don't come any more personal, and you have an unquestioned right to your own.

There are both gender-neutral and gender-specific taboos about anal pleasure that must be overcome to even begin our deliberations. These have been reinforced for so long, from such a young age, at such a deep level, and by such draconian methods that it takes some daring to find out for yourself what's actually relevant to you and what's not. For starters, you must acknowledge what, exactly, your beliefs and as-

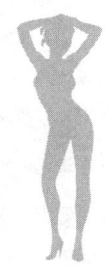

sumptions about butts and butt play are. Here are some typical knee-jerk (or sphincter-clench) reactions about butts: They're dirty, butt play or butt sex is "unnatural," butt play or butt sex is "homo/queer/gay/weak/effeminate," butts are "exit only," and butt play or butt sex is "immoral." Those who hold these opinions rarely examine them, but they run directly counter to my own observations.

Complicating understanding still further are contradictory attitudes that often lurk beneath the surface of such misconceptions. At the same time you may feel or believe some or all of these things, you may also be thinking, however guiltily, that butt sex might be sexy, hot, fun, nasty (in the playful sense), and transgressive and wishing that you could give it a try. It is the ever more elusive thrill of the forbidden in a gradually liberalizing society that, in my opinion, drives the current craze for anal-themed porn. I'm old enough to remember when a blow job was considered daring, and the human body has a limited number of openings. While debunking some myths about anal sex, I'll try to avoid stripping it of its naughtiness completely. If this helps any, Iraq's Grand Ayatollah Sistani tells us on his website that anal sex between men and women, while not forbidden, is still "highly discouraged," which represents the broad theological perspective of the great Abrahamic religions on the subject.

On to the debunking we go. Let's start with the notion of "dirty." Since solid waste is eliminated from the body via the anus, many believe that butts are "dirty" by default. This seems logical, and people don't often think to look beyond it. In fact, the anus and rectum are merely passageways for poop. As my friend Tristan Taormino puts it, "The rectum is not a storage facility." If you maintain a healthy diet, with plenty of fiber and water, your bowel movements will be regular and complete, and there will be little, if any, solid matter left at the business end of your guts most of the time. Bear in mind that anal sex and anal play of most kinds involve only the lower eight inches of your thirty-plus feet of intestinal plumbing, and keeping the relevant plumbing in good working order isn't particularly difficult. All that's needed for a butt to be play-clean is a little rinse with water (details to come, ready or not) and the use of a baby wipe or warm, soapy wash-cloth on the external sphincter. A freshly washed anus is just as clean as a patch of skin a few inches away on a butt cheek you wouldn't hesitate to kiss. Remember what they told me in nursing school: There's nothing that can't be washed off, so relax, already.

Now, does this mean that there is no chance of a random encounter with some small quantity of fecal matter despite your best efforts? I'm tempted to quote a popular saying about "what" happens in life, but, as the saying implies, you needn't overreact if and when it does. The short version: If you want to explore butt play and butt sex, you must get over your fear of shit. The most common bacterium it contains— *E. coli*—can be hazardous to your health in the wrong place at the wrong time in the wrong amount, but I wouldn't rate its toxicity any-where near that of, say, botulinum, which many of us pay to have in-jected into our foreheads.

Women can have a particularly hard time with the notion of butt sex because we're supposed to be clean, delicate, dainty creatures made out of sugar and spice and everything nice, and our physiologies tend to be inconveniently messy as it is. Butt play and butt sex are also raunchy and animalistic by nature, and many women think of that kind of sexuality as distinctly masculine. Moreover, early anal experi-mentation tends to be initiated by men, who may not know much about the subject either, often with unpleasant results. One bad poke can put a woman off butt play for years. But it remains true that, in order to

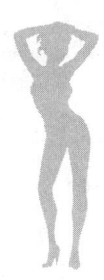

enjoy butt play, a woman has to jettison her notions of "propriety" and "ladylike" behavior, as there is little that is more primal than butt sex.

It's also a common notion that butt play or butt sex is *unnatural*. I'm never sure exactly what that word means in this context, since many higher mammals engage in anal sex, and humans have been doing it, literally, since before we began standing upright. How common a behavior must become to be considered "natural" is difficult to quantify. I suppose that if you believe sex is mainly or only for procreation, then butt play or butt sex might be considered "against nature" (though nature's intent in making it so common and enjoyable would thus be a bit mysterious), but if you view sex primarily as a means of reproduction, I'm a little curious as to why you're reading this book in the first place. At the risk of trespassing on the turf of those whose job it is to parse such imponderables, I believe that no consensual, mutually pleasurable activity should be forbidden between lovers. Labeling anal pleasure "unnatural" is generally an attempt by social and religious institutions to keep you from trying it for yourself. I think you're capable of making your own decision here, don't you? This is your ass we're talking about.

When the topic turns to butt play with men in the recipient role, we slam up against the wall of homophobia full force. The notion that all receptive anal sex among men is proof positive of gay orientation is a myth of awesome power and reach. The social oppression surrounding it is so brutal that the vast majority of men of all orientations are denied this locus of pleasure altogether and risk being beaten within an inch of their lives should they bring up the topic among other men. I'm sure you won't be surprised to discover that I harbor no disapproval whatsoever of actual gayness, do not regard it as any threat to anything worth defending, and think that those who do should just get over it. On the contrary, I believe that straight men can learn a lot from their gay brothers on how to pursue full-body pleasure, the likes of which they've likely never known.

As any gay man can attest, liking butt play doesn't make a man gay. Sexual orientation is a matter of partner preference, not behavior. If you, as a man, prefer to have sex with women, regardless of the specific activities involved, you are not gay, so there. However, if you are open to anal stimulation, you are an uninhibited sensualist and damn lucky. Unlike your insecure pals at the gym, you have access to additional sources of mind-blowing orgasms. I find it poignantly sad that so many men who would like to pursue anal pleasure but can't get past the social barriers against it cover their uneasiness with homophobic banter to the detriment of all, especially themselves. Once again, I advise listening to the wisdom of the body and advising others to kiss your ass or that of whomever they would rather. Just remember that if you see a woman when you look back over your shoulder while it's happening, you're no less straight than you would have been had you entertained the fantasy and never acted on it.

What about the view, held by both genders, that butt sex is wrong because butts are "exit only"? Anatomically speaking, colons are simply tubes, and tubes go both ways. When anal sex is practiced sensibly and safely, there is no anatomical factor that makes it inherently more difficult, dangerous, or destructive to the human body than other forms of sex. The common fear that anal penetration will eventually lead to a permanent loosening of the sphincter, incontinence, hemorrhoids, or other irreversible damage to the plumbing involved has much more to do with what goes on in people's heads than in regions farther south. Sphincter muscles are naturally equipped to dilate and contract repeatedly and will continue to do so normally regardless of direction, if treated with reasonable care and consideration. Indeed, regular anal

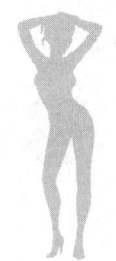

play both relaxes and strengthens internal muscle tissue and contributes to healthy bowel function.

In the end, as it were, the issue comes down to buggery and how you feel about it. Letting go of anal taboos is a task you must undertake for yourself, for your own reasons, and in your own good time. If and when you're ready to do so, you'll find the physical obstacles far less daunting than the psychological barriers you've already overcome.

Preparation: His and Hers, Mind and Body

In X-rated videos, butt sex happens by magic. One minute the players are fucking conventionally, and the next he's in her ass without so much as a pause for reflection, much less lube. This magic is called editing, and it doesn't work in real life. I shudder to contemplate how many people think that this is the norm and try it that way at home. Performers are professionals who are hired to do a certain thing at which they have had much practice. And even for the pros, anal sex requires proper advance planning. Before the scene even gets started, she's done her pre–butt-sex routine and is ready to go. The players have worked out the positions they're going to do, and the director knows how many minutes of footage are needed for each. Any difficulties that might ensue are excised from the final product, so it all looks perfectly smooth and effortless. Your mileage may vary—considerably. You may eventually reach the level of easy expertise you see in videos, but getting there will take dedication on your part and that of your partner or partners.

Unlike our genitals, anuses provide few clues from the outside. They can be pigmented from pale pink to dark brown, and the size of the aperture has no correlation to how much or how little prior attention they've received. Variations in appearance are largely genetic. The characteristic pucker enables the anus to open for bowel movements and then close up tightly. Anuses are remarkably elastic. The butt of a person under anesthesia can easily accommodate the hand of a surgeon, with the patient none the worse on awakening. However, the most important thing for novice anal players to understand is that butts are not "stretched" open. Rather, they are coaxed into relaxation. Their internal mechanisms cannot be rushed or compelled into cooperation.

Directly inside the external sphincter lie the anal canal and the internal sphincter. The anal canal is about two to three inches long, and the nerve endings concentrated there are extremely dense. How dense? When I first got into regular, pleasurable anal play, I likened the sensation of internal stimulation to having my clit elongated, hollowed out, and tickled from the inside. As we've already established that a clit contains as much nerve tissue as the head of a penis, you get the idea. Beyond the second sphincter is the rectum, which is as far as all but the most determined butt players will ever go, or need to. The rectum is delicate but isn't as sensitively wired as the anus itself. As a rule, it can detect sharp, deep, or pokey sensations but not gentle ones. Every anal canal is tilted a bit differently, none going in a straight line, which is another reason to proceed with caution when playing with butts. Each has an internal roadway that needs to be mapped by careful exploration. Like vaginas, butts expand and "balloon" when stimulated and will straighten slightly in the process, but only to a certain point. And, unlike vaginas, rectums are internally uniform, without all the folds, pockets, and terrain features with which the former come equipped, which is one reason why anal sex feels so different from vaginal intercourse for both the giving and receiving partners. There is a crucial dif-

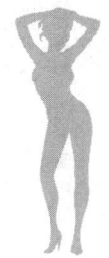

ference between genders in the construction of the lower colon, which is the location of the prostate gland in men. An egg-shaped bump just beyond the internal sphincter, it is as responsive as a woman's G-spot and is wired directly to a man's genital receptors. Many men find that stimulation of the prostate produces the most intense orgasms of which they are capable, which is reason enough to become familiar with it.

While anal anatomy isn't particularly complex, its operation is subtle, delicate, and unpredictable. It requires a degree of awareness and concentration to become a source of reliable enjoyment and satisfaction. There is no faking it through the anal experience. Your butt is incapable of lying. If it's not entirely happy, it will let you know, and no amount of "training" will make it receptive to clumsy handling. Your first attempts to inspire a positive response from it may be compromised by some of the emotional factors we've already discussed or by the unfamiliarity of the new physical sensations. Don't be discouraged if your initial anal-sex encounters prove a bit daunting. The rewards are well worth working for.

Even though I only have full anal intercourse a few times a month, I include some anal stimulation every time I have sex, so butt cleaning is a regular part of my preplay routine. As a result, I can make love fully confident that there will be no messy surprises for either of us. I've also come to enjoy the ritual of putting myself in the headspace for anal adventure to whatever degree it will actually proceed. What's needed: gloves, lube (we'll discuss lube options in detail shortly), an anal bulb syringe, and privacy in the bathroom. Fill the syringe (available at a good adult store) with cool or warm water and set it within easy reach. Put on a pair of latex gloves, sit on the toilet, and lube up the middle finger of your nondominant hand. Slide the finger into your anus to the third knuckle and relax your muscles as you exhale, pulling yourself open just a little. Using that finger as a guide (to avoid damaging the delicate tissue), slide the nozzle of the syringe alongside of it and then remove your finger.

Remaining relaxed, use both hands to squeeze the water out of the syringe, flushing out any solid matter that may be present. You'll probably pee, too, and that's fine. Repeat up to three times, always relubricating your finger before inserting it, and you should expel nothing but clear water. If things are still messy, your butt is just not in the mood and will have the evening off. Pull the gloves off inside out and discard before washing your hands and using a washcloth or baby wipe to clean up your crotch and butt. Now you're ready for anything, from a gloved thumb to your favorite toy to an actual penis. I've got the whole exercise down to five minutes.

Some regular anal players prefer to prepare with a full enema, rinsing out their entire colons a couple of hours prior to whatever enjoyable activities they have planned. I'm not against this practice per se, as I know many people find it pleasing in itself and feel some added sense of security when it comes to cleanliness thereafter. However, as we've established that only the bottom few inches of the lower colon's S curve are likely to be involved, enemas aren't really necessary for hygiene purposes, and their effects can be unpredictable. Depending on how soon they're administered after a meal, for instance, they can actually precipitate a more rapid descent of the intestine's contents than would otherwise occur and make things messier rather than neater. They can also induce cramping and, if done too frequently, cause dehydration, leading to drier, more vulnerable membranes.

If you regard enemas as a must, keep them simple. I would avoid the prepackaged variety if it contains any soaps or chemicals and stick with plain water, warmed as closely as possible to body temperature.

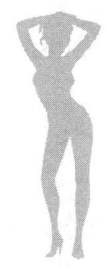

There's a wide range of specialized gear available through sex-goods purveyors for true enema fanciers, but the ordinary combination douche/enema kit sold at your local drugstore is more than adequate for simple cleansing purposes. And under no circumstances would I recommend adding alcohol or other intoxicants to the mix, as they are far more readily absorbed through the intestinal wall than when consumed orally, and even small amounts can produce toxic reactions ranging from merely unpleasant to downright fatal.

Too Good to Hurry

So, just how do I approach my partner's butt or how does my husband approach mine? With absolute respect and patience, which builds the necessary confidence to push on. The recipient must know that you will never, EVER, move to penetration of even the least intrusive kind without explicit consent or invitation. You earn trust by being trustworthy, and you can easily ruin months' worth of practice in one hasty, inconsiderate moment. The simple truth to keep in mind is this: Butts must be coaxed and seduced each and every time, no matter what happened on the previous occasion. No one "gets" ass. You must earn ass by learning to "speak ass," as one of my girlfriends puts it. My husband and I have an understanding: He can play with my butt whenever *he* wants, but he can't fuck it until *it* wants. His job is to get it in the mood, and my job is to relax and let it happen. Some days, a butt plug is all that's happening, and on other days, I really need him to fuck me there. Let your butt be your guide, and you'll be fine.

Our initial reaction to anything near our butts is usually to clench, so the first priority of the recipient of any butt play is relaxation. Breathe into the clench as you relax the muscles. At first, you'll be able to relax for, oh, a half second or less, as the sensations rush in and whatever negative conditioning you've absorbed attempts to assert itself. Pause, breathe, and relax again. As you become more comfortable with the intensity of anal stimulation, you'll be able to relax for longer and longer moments. I started with being able to relax for a half second, but now I can stay comfortable with my ass in action for half an hour, and I don't consider myself an exceptionally anal person. Some will obviously find this comes more easily than others will, and I admit to a bit of wonderment at those who can accommodate large objects quickly and easily, but there is no right or wrong here and no competition to see whose ass is the most elastic. Take your time and don't fault yourself for responses you can't command.

A good warm-up can begin with simply pulling the butt cheeks apart during foreplay or vaginal sex. This gentle stretching of the skin is more erotic than you might expect. Pull and release as your partner winks his or her anus, then pull again. As with pussy play, release when the butt is clenched and spread again when the butt is relaxed. Moving on from there, try rubbing a lubed or spit-wet thumb over the anus itself in small circles, noting the response; a rub-rub-rest/rub-rub-rest rhythm is very effective. A couple may stay at this stage of anal play for weeks or months, as the sensations become first familiar and then sensual. This is when trust is earned and teamwork developed.

Often, initial penetration comes as the tip of the thumb slides in to the first knuckle during an especially happy wink. If it does, don't press your luck by pushing in deeper. As we say in show business, "Leave 'em wanting more." This is the only time it's okay to touch the anus without gloves (if your nails are short and smooth, that is), as you're not going in deep enough to get dirty.

If you've done your presex butt-cleaning routine, your anus is clean

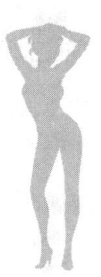

enough to lick, which is called "rimming" in the vernacular and "anni-lingus" in the Latin. I'm here to say it's fun to do and it feels wonderful to receive, once you've moved past your "butt-equals-dirty" inhibitions. While deep rimming that involves actual tongue penetration of the anus runs some risk of bacterial exposure, external rimming is safe and fun, and neither men nor women should deny themselves the en-joyment it affords. I'm always surprised when men resist my efforts to please them in this way (although by now I suppose I shouldn't be), as if taking satisfaction in having their asses licked by a woman somehow puts their gender orientation in doubt. Licking, kissing, and nuzzling are all good moves. If a man will let me, I'll rim him and stroke his cock simultaneously. Those secure enough to allow this report that it ranks among the greatest of erotic delights. Rimming is also an excellent segue to anal penetration, subtly alerting the anal nerves to the possi-bility of additional pleasures to come.

The tools you need for basic butt play are simple, starting with a good lube. Unlike pussies, butts do not lubricate themselves, and tastes in lube vary widely. I prefer a thick, water-based gel such as ID Glide for its greater viscosity and for the added protection of my internal tis-sues provided by its slightly heavier density. However, many experi-enced anal players, who want the maximum sensation combined with the highest degree of slickness, choose thinner silicone formulations like Eros, which have the advantage of remaining "wet" indefinitely without evaporating or turning tacky. I strongly advise against any lube that contains a numbing agent. Though such products promise to make anal play easier, in fact, they merely deaden the sensation and increase the odds of doing damage to fragile interior terrain. Pain is a warning from your body that something isn't right, and any product that silences that alarm puts you at risk of injury. Read the label of any product carefully to be certain that no local anesthetic is present before purchasing any new brand. Over time, you'll find your own optimal product by experimentation. Different lubes work better with different toys, so you may develop a small collection of butt-friendly lubes, the better to mix and match.

Whatever formulations you choose, remember to use them liberally and repeatedly. Insufficient lubrication is the greatest single cause of anal-sex discomfort. Anal play is much more focused on penetration than friction, which is almost never enjoyable. The only caveat to the rule of No Such Thing as Too Much Lube concerns hygiene: Some leakage of lube is likely to occur in the course of an anal-play session, and if it finds its way into an unprotected vagina, bacterial contamination may result in a thoroughly unpleasant infection requiring medical treatment. So keep those wipes handy!

On a related note, you'll also want to invest in some latex gloves, now available in virtually every drugstore and sex-toy shop. They'll take a bit of getting used to at first, but once you find the right size and the minimal thickness necessary, you'll come to appreciate the way they keep your hands clean for other uses. Think of them as "hand condoms." After lubing up a butt, they can be discarded, and your clean hands can be used to stimulate other parts without fear of cross-contamination. Don't be stingy with them; once they've done their job, they're to be discarded and replaced with new ones when your fingers return to anal activities of any sort.

Before serious consideration can be given to inserting a live penis into an anus, a butt plug or other toy is a vital intermediate instrument. When we get to our chapter on toys, I'll go into greater detail regarding the options available, but a quick visit to your local sex-goods emporium will cause you to marvel at the inventiveness of the human

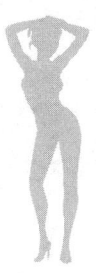

imagination when it comes to devising implements for opening asses. Butt plugs range from tiny ticklers barely larger than a finger to shudder-inducing battering rams the thickness of fire hydrants. Clearly, you'll want to start small. The only absolute requisite for a proper butt toy is a widely flared base. Straight, cylindrical objects, while perfectly fine for vaginal use, can easily slide into a well-greased anus and migrate upward, leading to anxious moments at best and embarrassing trips to the emergency room at worst. Every ER intern has war stories of inappropriate objects removed from suffering butts by means you don't even want to contemplate.

After you get home from your shopping spree with your bag of lubes, gloves, and plugs, you need to contain your excitement long enough to master the simple but critical skill of inserting an anal toy correctly. I have my partner turn onto one hip and pull open a cheek, or lie on his or her back with knees open. It's important that the person whose ass is to be plugged be able to completely relax, the better to focus attention. Of course, by the time we pay attention to the butt, there's been plenty of pleasurable play already, so the engine's revving nicely. With a male partner, his cock may or may not deflate as his attention is directed elsewhere, and that's okay.

For the first six months that I was practicing, I needed to touch my clit while my husband (who was already very fluent in ass-speak) worked my butt, as it kept the sensation from becoming too focused and intense. Keeping my clit in the mix made the sensation "bigger" by combining the anal and the clitoral sensations, which, in turn, enabled me to keep my anus relaxed for longer. I no longer need to do that, but it really helped in the beginning. For many women, clit stimulation will always be a vital component in the formula for sublime anal enjoyment. The two certainly work well. Likewise, attention to the penis during any kind of male butt play should never be stinted. Connecting anal and genital sensations is one of the keys to back-door satisfaction.

I glove up both hands and apply lube to my finger. Gently placing my finger against my partner's anus, I press forward a little, pushing the lube inside. I'll do this two or three times before I actually try to insert my finger farther. As with pussy play, when the butt tightens, I stop moving, and when it relaxes, I'll tickle lightly again. With butts, three movements are needed, sometimes separately and sometimes in tandem. One is the classic in-and-out movement of the finger. When you get a good rhythm going, you may be able to slide your entire finger in and out easily. The second movement is a massagelike circling of the sphincter rings to encourage them to relax. Apply pressure with your finger until the butt clenches. Stop pressing, and in a second or two the butt will relax and you can press against the muscle again. The goal here is to increase the ratio of relaxed intervals to clenched intervals. I encourage my partners to masturbate while I do this to keep the wires between anal and genital sensation hot. The third movement is tickling, making tiny "coochie-coo" movements with your fingertip just beyond the external sphincter, where the nerve bundles are thickest, or beyond the internal ones, which also feels great. Combining these moves, while never a complete guarantee of the desired loosening, will bring about the most predictably desirable responses.

When you can easily insert a full finger and tickle and press without discomfort, you can enjoy the intimate invasiveness of massaging your partner's tailbone from the inside. If your partner is deriving the intended benefits, he or she will start to fuck your finger back and make deep, guttural, primal noises that are distinct from those common to vaginal sex. This is your cue to increase the rate and/or pres-

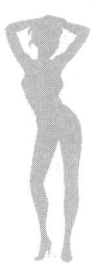

sure and/or depth of the stimulation. With enough practice, you'll learn when it's time to try two fingers, obviously doubling the intensity. Once two fingers are easy for your partner, a toy or plug will be no problem. Remember, getting from "Oh, I'd like to try it" to "Yeah, baby, fuck my ass!" can take months to a year. The only "goal" should be pleasure and not the ability to fit something in your butt that you saw in a video. Start small and work up gradually. Remember that the anal experience is more about girth than depth, as most anal sensation is concentrated in those first few inches, so gradually increasing the width of your toys is a higher priority than going for deeper probes. Once the plug is inserted, use a baby wipe to remove all traces of lube (we mustn't be messy while we are being dirty, after all), pull the gloves off inside out, and you're ready for whatever is next, which is strictly up to the two of you.

A butt plug offers other opportunities for enjoyment beyond its function of opening the anus for further attention. A woman, for example, can be fucked vaginally with a modestly sized plug in place, tightening her pussy and providing her partner with an intriguing internal pressure point to rub against while she experiences some of the delightful fullness of double penetration. External application of a vibrator or other clitoral stimulation or insertion of a vaginal toy at the same time can produce spectacularly orgasmic results. My husband and I often use the plug in conjunction with other sexual activities as an enhancement, with no intention of proceeding to actual butt fucking.

However, if anal intercourse is to be the main attraction, the preliminary use of a toy is primarily a means of helping the sphincters relax and the body become accustomed to the sensation of anal penetration. As such, it should remain in place long enough to become comfortable.

It can be manipulated or remain stationary, according to taste, but if it fails to produce the desired loosening effect and remains an intrusive presence, the signs are not right for anal sex, which should be deferred to another day. The fact that a plug or other toy is a delight on one occasion and a literal pain in the ass on another merely demonstrates once again that butts are fickle and moody and cannot be willed into cooperation.

Adjusting Your Attitude Before Your Anatomy Does It for You

It will take a lot of practice—a great deal of hard pounding in Cirque du Soleil positions—before you can have anal intercourse as we do on-screen, if you ever get that far. Fucking an ass is not like fucking a pussy, and you can't go about it in the same way. Think of you, your partner, and your butts as a team: You've got to learn to work together and to read each other's signals in order to make your plays smoothly. No rushing. No ego. No emulating porn folks. Anal injuries from too much friction, not enough lube, not enough warm-up, improper technique, the wrong toy, or ignoring bodily signals are no laughing matter. The worst can require surgery to correct, which will not endear you to your sweetheart.

Between butt plugs and butt fucking, I suggest graduating to the use of dildos. My own anal education progressed from a finger to a small dildo to two fingers, then to a medium dildo (about 80 percent of the size of my husband's cock), and finally to his actual penis. I still find a need for continuing education. If it's been a while between butt fuckings, I'll go back to the medium dildo for a few minutes before attempting to take a cock again. It feels good to be stuffed like that, and while

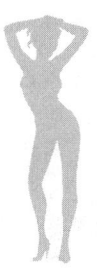

we're working up to the main event, he can slide the dildo in and out in tandem with his pussy fucking for an amazing dual-socket sensation.

Having something in my butt makes his cock feel bigger and my pussy feel tighter. The creative use of butt plugs can go a long way toward resolving any "size differential" a couple may experience, since the plugs come in any size you can think of. I have a favorite plug—bullet-shaped and made of stainless steel with a flexible shaft—that I use almost every time we make love to create a sensation my husband and I both enjoy. As you progress toward actual anal intercourse, keep in mind all you've learned about breathing, relaxing, and communicating.

While engaged in these activities, it's extremely important to avoid cross-contamination between butts and pussies. One wrong poke with a finger, toy, or cock can produce an infection that will put your female partner out of commission for ten days. Avoid touching her pussy with a glove, toy, or penis that's had prior anal contact, and make sure no lube drips from her anus to her vagina. That's why I suggest doing the preliminaries with the woman on her back rather than on her knees, as gravity can undermine your best intentions. If you suspect such accidental contamination has occurred, take a break while she washes her pussy with warm, soapy water. Obviously, during anal intercourse you may NOT "double-dip," going from ass to pussy. Nurse Nina says: "It doesn't matter that you may have seen performers do this in a video. They shouldn't have, and the editor probably cut out the trip to the clinic that followed." I know it would feel good, but the enjoyment would be far less enduring than the consequences. If she needs something in her pussy while you're in her butt, she can use her fingers or a toy of choice.

Counterintuitive though it may seem, beginners often find anal sex easiest in the missionary position. The active partner kneeling between the receptive partner's legs has good visual contact with the relevant anatomy and its owner. Eye contact is helpful in reading subtle signals of pleasure and/or discomfort and inspires trust and confidence. If the receptive partner is female, her clit will be accessible—a definite plus. When I'm wearing a strap-on or using a handheld toy and fucking a guy, he can relax, and we can play with his cock and balls. Some men remain rock hard while they're getting it in the butt, while others lose their erections as their attentions, fantasies, and energies are redirected.

Some women absolutely require vaginal stimulation to enjoy anal penetration, and having her pussy available to her own fingers or favorite toy is a must. Use a smaller, squishier dildo than you would otherwise, as things will be tighter than usual. The obvious drawback to missionary anal sex is the tendency of the anus to tilt downward. This can be compensated for by placing a pillow under the buttocks and raising the legs in the air. Lying on the edge of a couch or a big, overstuffed chair with the ass hanging over the edge just a little also provides a good angle for penetration.

"Spooning" is a very comfy way to take it in the butt, facilitating full-body caresses and convenient genital access (remember to keep those hands clean!). This works particularly well for a man with a long cock who is ass fucking a female partner. She's free to wiggle against him all she wants as she simultaneously humps him and uses a vibrator on her clit if desired. Be careful during insertion, as it's easy here to miss and hit her pussy, so have her cover it with her hand during the initial anal entry.

If a man sits in a big chair, "lap dancing" takes on a whole new meaning as his partner lowers herself onto his cock while facing away. She can control the angle and depth of penetration, and he gets a great view. (The sounds I make in this position are the most primal of all, as

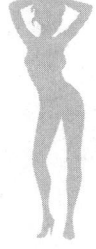

I can get him in very deep, which produces extremely intense sensations.) If he's propped up against the headboard of a bed, she can kneel over his lap and sit on him, facing in either direction, depending on which position is more comfortable.

The classic positions for anal intercourse, regardless of the recipient's gender, are hands-and-knees doggy or standing while bent over. If the "catcher" is female, it's a good idea to hold a baby wipe over her pussy during insertion so that a fresh application of lube isn't squeegeed off a dick or dildo and down onto her pussy. Start slow, as you wait for the butt to relax and accommodate. Soon enough you'll be rocking along. If your partner even hints at needing more lube, stop instantly and regrease all components. Since the strongest sensations are felt in the first inches of the rectum, there's something sweetly nasty about multiple insertions during butt sex, so try to think of the necessary lube stops as ramping up the action rather than slowing it down. Doggy style is particularly effective for strap-on work with a male partner, if comfortable arrangements can be made for the usual height differential. Pay attention to his noises as you massage his prostate with the toy. He may—or may not—be able to come this way. Do it for as long as it feels good and then move on to something else.

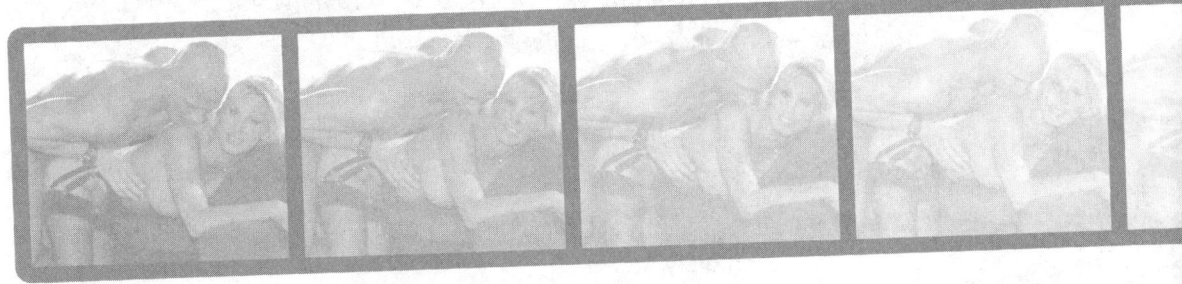

BOFFO BUTT PLEASERS

1 • *Lube, lube, lube.* You cannot have too much lube. Ditto gloves. Ditto baby wipes.

2 • *Take your time.* Why rush a good thing?

3 • *Patience will be rewarded.* Treat your partner's butt as you would treat your own.

4 • *Butts can't lie.* If it's not in the mood, move on to something else.

5 • *For consistently good anal experiences, eat plenty of fiber and drink lots of water.* A healthy colon is a happy and receptive colon.

6 • *Start small, with fingers and toys and brief play periods.* You'll work up to the main event in due course.

7 • *Stay focused.* Anal sex requires more care than other penetrative play. Stay alert for possible discomfort or cross-contamination.

8 • *Know when to quit.* Anuses, no matter how well prepped, are generally less suited to long, hard fucking than other parts.

BUTT BUNGLES

1 • *No guilt-tripping your partner into going along with butt play,* unless you're trying to engineer a breakup.

2 • *No matter how horny you are, do not short the warm-up.* You'll get less of what you want in the long run.

3 • *No attempting to emulate professionals while you're still in train-ing.* Keep the gymnastics (and the Louisville slugger) in your mind's eye.

4 • *Don't grit it out.* If your ass signals distress, stop what you're do-ing immediately.

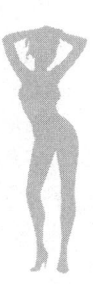

5 • *Don't put anything into a butt not specifically designed for that purpose.* That soda bottle only seems like a good idea.

6 • *Don't be drunk or high.* This increases the odds of mishaps you'll both regret later.

7 • *Don't flip out if things get a bit messy.* It can happen even with the most conscientious prior planning. Just clean up and move on without making a fuss.

8 • *No switching of orifices without pausing for a hygiene stop.* What lives in the ass needs to stay in the ass. Mouths and pussies are no place for *E. coli.*

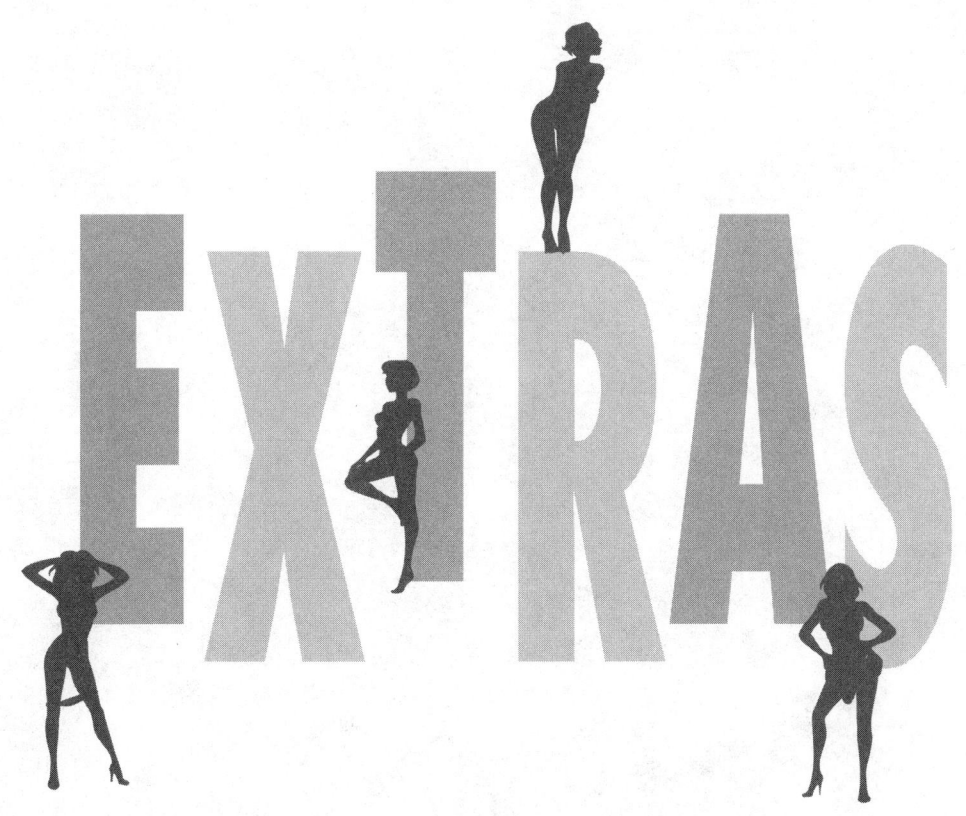

Chapter 11

TOYS:
PUTTING TECHNOLOGY TO WORK

oderns like ourselves prefer to think we invented the world whole in our own lifetimes, especially when it comes to something as important as sex. Looking at the dizzying array of widgets, gadgets, and gizmos to be found in any contemporary sex-goods emporium, it would be easy enough to conclude that the science of creating pleasure-enhancing devices for lovers is an entirely recent phenomenon. The historic record tells us something quite different. Archaeologists have found penis substitutes made of wood, bone, ivory, and polished stone that date to prehistoric times. Ben-wa balls for vaginal insertion and hanging baskets for feminine-superior intercourse positions date to ancient China. Recipes for unguents, lotions, and potions meant to enhance sexual pleasure appear on Egyptian papyruses, and both Greek and Roman pottery and frescoes depict the use of strap-on dildos by men and women alike. Marble cock rings turn up in the digs of Pompeii.

This is hardly surprising; human beings are inventive by nature, and their ingenuity tends to focus on those things that give pleasure, either in the form of material rewards or sensual satisfaction. Man the Toolmaker has, from the dawn of sentience, looked to his environment for means of augmenting his powers, increasing his abilities, and satisfying his desires. Few motivations to invention could be more obvious or compelling than the urge to intensify the rewards of sexuality.

If the earliest examples of sex toys are quaint, simple, and obvious in design and function, the dawn of the industrial revolution and the age of invention brought quantum leaps in the application of technology to both the facilitation of sexual expression and its obstruction. As science and medicine began to examine the physical mechanisms of sexuality, competing theories arose as to what constituted healthy and natural sexual behavior and what did not, with technologies to both ends arising simultaneously. Crude chastity belts, mainly meant to secure the rights of primogeniture, gave way to cruel "anti-self-abuse" devices meant to discourage masturbation with everything from spiked harnesses to electroshock contraptions. As always, however, attempts to inhibit sexual pleasure invariably accompany efforts to intensify it or at least to bring it under some semblance of voluntary control.

What I consider the first modern sex toy combines both motivations in a technological advance that has proved far more durable and widespread in its application than its inventors could ever have imagined—the electric vibrator. Electric vibrators were originally developed as labor-saving devices for doctors who, well into the nineteenth century, were expected to manually manipulate the genitalia of their female

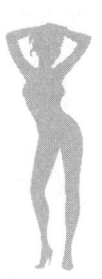

patients in order to "cure" hysteria. The symptoms of "hysteria" (derived from the Greek *hysterikos,* meaning "of the womb") were eerily similar to those of chronic sexual frustration: sleeplessness, irritability, moodiness, pelvic congestion, and discomfort. The medical "cure" was to induce "hysterical paroxysm," aka sexual orgasm. Not too surprisingly, women of the more affluent classes had to visit their doctors regularly for such "cures," and, with that peculiar sensibility Victorians regarded as progressive, no one thought it odd in the slightest. Just as "self-abuse" was, for years, ferociously discouraged by the most extreme methods imaginable, the doctor's touch removed the stigma of animal lust. Doctors who didn't care for this aspect of private practice would train their nurses or midwives to perform the onerous procedure for them, as it could take an hour or more for a single patient to achieve her "cure." With the advent of the electric vibrator, a doctor could "treat" many more women in a single day. It wasn't long before these early, cumbersome prototypes began to make their way into the hands of ordinary folk, and by the early years of the last century, they were available through the Sears-Roebuck catalogue.

If the technological revolution brought us the basic mechanical means to extend our natural capabilities as lovers, it took the sexual revolution another fifty years to free our imaginations in creating devices and artifacts for the intensification of erotic pleasure. The proliferation of sex toys since the great sexual awakening of the late twentieth century has been nothing less than staggering. We now find ourselves confronted with dildos of every size, shape, color, and construction; simulated vaginas made of "lifelike" polymer plastics; electrostimulation systems for both internal and external use by either gender; vibrators ranging from lipstick size to industrial strength; vacuum pumps for clits and dicks; automated fucking machines with interchangeable insertables;

specialized furniture to enable every imaginable sex position; and even creepily realistic, full-size, highly detailed fuck dolls upholstered in "cyberskin." Obviously, not all these inventions are equally valuable in shaping a fulfilling sex life, but it's worth your time to get to know what's out there, make informed choices as sophisticated sex-toy consumers, and, most important, learn how to integrate your acquisitions into your individual sex lives for maximum benefit.

Sex toys have come a long way since their advertisement and sale were barely legal (and in a few backward states, they're still prohibited), so if you've ever had a less-than-satisfying experience with a sex toy, now's the time to replace that sad memory with a hot one.

Why Toys?

When it comes to sex toys, I've found people fall into roughly four camps: "the more the merrier," "never thought of them," "they skeeve me out," and "why?" Sex toys are merely objects designed to promote erotic pleasure. Think of them as tools for the bedroom, just as your fancy food processor is a tool for the kitchen, your power drill is a tool for the workshop, and your deluxe vacuum cleaner is a tool for your living room. Use them to intensify or extend enjoyment, experiment with new sensations, provide that extra stimulation needed for orgasmic fulfillment, or lessen the labor involved in satisfying our partners and ourselves. When you become sufficiently comfortable with your own sexuality to seek out new ways of expanding your enjoyment of it, the use of toys is as natural to your experimental progression as any lovemaking technique you might acquire.

A sex toy can be as simple as a swatch of fur or velvet used to stroke

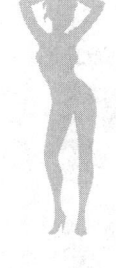

bare skin or as complex as a mechanical penetration device costing in the low four figures. Indeed, as long as they won't hurt tender flesh and can be cleaned completely or covered with a condom, many common household objects can be and are used as sex toys. Many people's early experiments with toy play involve hairbrush handles, washing machines, and even power tools. However, dedicated erotic explorers soon move on to more specialized gear, quickly discovering that quality made-for-sex toys aren't cheap, with a single dildo or vibrator costing as much as a hundred dollars.

Almost without exception, you get what you pay for. I have a lot of toys, expensive and not so, that looked intriguing in the store but failed to deliver the goods when I tried them on my actual anatomy at home. Some of them have gone to appreciative users who found them more enjoyable than I did, while others still sit, forlorn, in a box at the back of my closet, waiting to be adopted. However, my somewhat costly product research has been well worth it, as I use the toys I like many times a month, and I've had many of them for years. Once you find the particular item that works for you, you'll never wonder again why people bother with sex toys.

What's in the Box?

Vibrators are manufactured in a vast array of shapes, sizes, and levels of power and effectiveness. Many women, myself included, need vibrators in order to come easily, more than once or at all, and these are often the first toys an individual or couple will acquire. There are three basic types: battery-operated, rechargeable, and plug-in. Of the battery-operated versions, some are tiny, using watch batteries, while others take three D cells, making them on the heavy side. Some vibrators are designed to be inconspicuous, the better to slide in between two bodies fucking, while others require substantial room to maneuver. There are gloves with little vibrators at the tip of each finger as well as individual fingertip vibrating units that can fit most places. There are even small vibrators that attach to a person's tongue! Some battery-operated or rechargeable toys are beautiful modern sculptures that can be left on the bedside table as decoration without your mother ever suspecting their true purposes. Many absolutely need to be kept out of sight to avoid awkward questions, knowing smirks, or raised eyebrows. Some battery-operated or rechargeable toys are designed for external stimulation only and are smooth and ovoid or have pubic bone–cupping curves, the better to tickle your clit. Others are molded for internal stimulation as they buzz—the classic "vibrating dildo."

Battery-operated toys have more range than corded toys but can lose power at the most awkward moments or lack enough juice for your needs. They're more portable than corded toys, of course, for those of you who want to take your fun on the road or to a picnic. But if you're a woman who needs strong stimulation in order to come, a battery-operated toy of any size may not send you over the edge, although it may serve to keep you at it in a delicious fashion. A clever partner can use a comparatively low-power device to tease you unmercifully as a form of foreplay. And an exception to the battery-power-equals-weak-buzz paradigm is the so-called "pocket rocket," which gets an amazing amount of zing out of one double A. Also, some battery vibes are even water resistant, though I've never tested this feature myself. This could certainly make bath time more fun.

Some popular battery-operated dildos have all sorts of bells and whistles and rotate or pulsate as they vibrate or have little beads

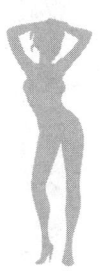

trapped behind flexible membranes designed to stimulate the friction-sensitive outer portion of the vaginal vault. These often include little waggly bits of silicone that oscillate to stimulate the clit. They're usually costly products imported from Japan (where ordinary dildos are still prohibited but fantastic examples of industrial design are common-place) and are, in my experience at least, more prone to failure than I am willing to accept in something so pricey. I also find those jigglesome out-croppings of humming silicone more annoying and irritating than stim-ulating. Of course, there are plenty of women out there who swear by their battery-operated twisty, waggly toys, so personal experimentation is the only reliable measure. One woman's orgasm is another woman's frustration; that's how you end up with toys you use only once.

My favorite plug-in vibrator is the Hitachi Magic Wand (or "Wanda," as a friend named hers), popularized nearly thirty years ago by the "godmother of masturbation," Betty Dodson. It's not an aesthetic tool, by any means, made as it is of white plastic, but, boy, does it do the job! It's very powerful and takes some getting used to, but it's also sturdy and hard to break, since it has only two speeds and a rugged internal motor. It takes a greedy girl indeed to burn one out, though I have been through a few over the years, which says more about me than about the Magic Wand. I keep one in my luggage, complete with the six-foot ex-tension cord, and one at home, as I forgot it once on a trip and resolved never to make that mistake again.

If the one hundred-twenty-volt AC vibe is too strong for you, fold a washcloth in halves or quarters and place it over your pubic bone be-fore applying the toy. Try moving your hips and keeping the toy still or keeping your hips still and subtly moving the toy. The clit is so richly endowed with nerve endings that even imperceptible movement of the vibrator produces great shifts in sensation. Try placing it against the

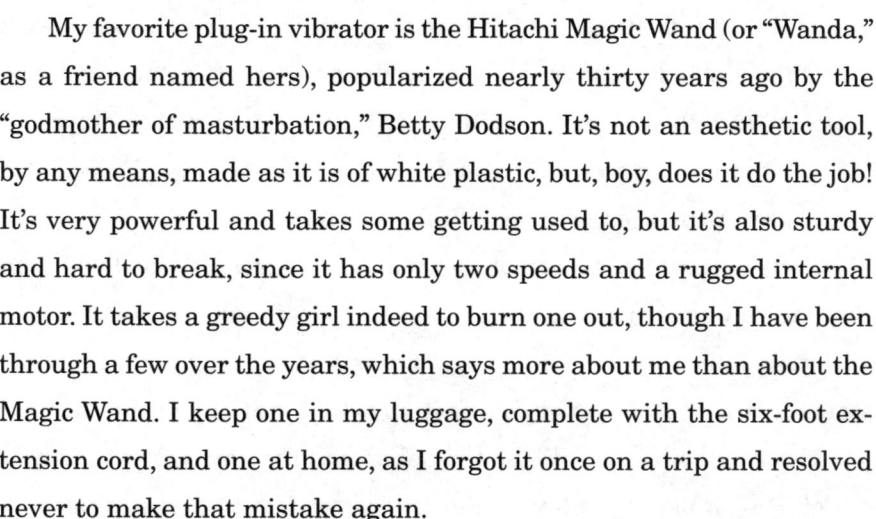

side of the shaft and rolling it five degrees or so, subtly using the motion to push the shaft to one side. Or roll it slowly down the top of the shaft. The secret with the wand is to move it more slowly than you might think necessary. You want to be able to feel every nerve fire off, and if you move the toy too quickly, you won't get the full effect. The pubic bone can act as an amplifier, causing the vibrations from direct stimulation to resonate through it behind the clit. Once you get this device in your hand, you're likely to try many variations with it until you find the combination of moves that works just right for you.

There's also a popular therapeutic toy, the Eroscillator™, that was designed with preorgasmic women in mind. It doesn't vibrate but rather oscillates back and forth thirty-six hundred times per minute. Of Swiss design, it's not as sturdy as the wand, but it's subtler and comes with interchangeable heads. The newest model now has attachments made of pussy-friendly silicone instead of hard plastic, which is an improvement. Many women swear by it, and, for what it's worth, the Eroscillator has earned some prestigious medical endorsements.

Some external-use-only vibrators are rechargeable, but I've found these to be weaker than I need. However, you or your lover may have a lower orgasmic threshold, and they may be fine under the right circumstances. Just don't forget to charge it up before that day in the country!

There are vibrating dildos that plug into the car cigarette-lighter outlet. Do not use these toys while driving, and, even if you're the passenger, don't distract the driver too much with your sexy show or you might have some embarrassing things to explain to the highway patrol, like how your car came to be wrapped around a tree with your panties down around your knees.

Dildos have come a long way in the past twenty thousand years, especially in the past two decades, thankfully. When I started in adult

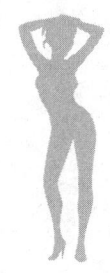

films, the dildos used in lesbian scenes were uniformly "flesh" colored (in those days, all flesh was assumed to be pink), made of some weird, hard plastic that didn't feel good next to tender parts no matter how much lube was used, and were almost always too big to actually fit any woman I knew. They were clearly designed by those who had never actually been close to a real pussy. Fortunately, female entrepreneurs set up shop in the sex-toy business not long after I began my career and started making dildos out of medical-grade silicone in all sizes, shapes, and colors.

Silicone is the best material for dildos, as it's sterilizable, can be cast in any desired shape or color, holds body heat, feels great on delicate membranes, and holds up well. (Some of my silicone toys are ten years old, at least.) There are only two things to keep in mind when playing with silicone dildos: Always use water-based lube, and don't bite them. If you use silicone-based lube with a silicone dildo, you must cover it with a condom, or the lube will ruin the surface of the toy and you'll be very bummed as well as out of a lot of money. And the tiniest tear in a silicone dildo will result in a clean break at that point, so no biting, and be careful with other kinds of hardware, such as strap-on harnesses. Silicone dildos come shaped like penises (eerily lifelike to rather abstractly phallic), dolphins, tongues, little goddesses or ears of corn, corkscrews, and other humorous or sacrilegious shapes that are as much novelty items as useful tools. They can also be designed for specific purposes, such as prostate or G-spot stimulation. Don't be surprised to find yourself giving them names to reflect their personalities.

Dildos can also be made of wood, glass (lovely and smooth, but you may need one thinner than you think to accommodate their inflexibility), Lucite, stone, horn, stainless steel, or bone. Dildos made of inflexible material are often oddly shaped, with curves, knobs, bumps, and bends, the better to tickle that perfect spot. These dildos don't lend themselves to use with harnesses, and many are equipped with handles for easier manipulation.

It's helpful to think of dildos as vaginal-massage devices rather than fake dicks, even though some of them are shaped like penises. This will help you move them more effectively inside yourself or your partner. The toy has no nerves and merely shoving it in and moving it around quickly won't convey the nuances of skin-to-skin contact you experience in real intercourse. Remember all those spots you found when you were lubing her up with your fingers? Slide the toy in slowly and seek out those same spots. Do you respond favorably to deep, slow, methodical pressure? Do you prefer shallower penetration with faster friction? Do you like the tip angled up, causing the base to stretch the introitus, or does it feel better when it's pressed into the back wall of the vagina? Simultaneous clitoral masturbation is an enhancement for most women, though a distraction to some.

When using a dildo on someone else, I usually start slow and will even hold the dildo still and let my female partner fuck it at her own speed and stroke, the better to gauge her needs. Try sliding it down toward her posterior fornix on the in-stroke and pulling it up to move past her G-spot on the out-stroke. More than simple friction (unless she's telling you to fuck her harder), it's vaginal manipulation that achieves the best results. Fucking a happy pussy with a toy feels like stirring a pot of thick oatmeal or pudding, or churning butter. It will close down around the base of the toy while making room for it to move internally. You'll be able to feel your partner's muscles grip and relax reflexively. It's good to be in shape, as I've worn out my arm with some of my more robust lovers.

Many couples like to play with strap-on dildos. While most often seen in use by two women in pornographic situations, strap-ons can be

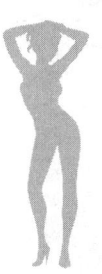

worn by men as well. Strap-on harnesses are worn around the hips to hold a dildo in place so the wearer can fuck his or her partner and keep his or her hands free for other things. They can be made from rubber, leather, vinyl, cloth, or a combination of these materials. There are two popular styles: the T-strap and the jock. The T-strap harness looks like a thong, with two hip straps and a third strap that passes between the legs and over the clit. The jock style has a waist strap as well as straps that pass around each thigh. This style of harness leaves the genitals of the wearer exposed for his or her pleasure. In both styles, the front of the harness contains the harness ring. This ring, made of rubber or metal, holds the base of the dildo, giving the wearer a firmer "erection." Most can be manipulated so that the ring fits the base of the toy snugly. Too big, and the toy simply falls out; too small, and the toy won't go in. It's important that the harness not be stretchy but fit as firmly as is comfortable. You want as little wiggle room as possible.

I found wearing a strap-on harness with a dildo in it super fun the very first time I tried it. Immediately, my hand went to my newly acquired "cock," and I wanted to stick it somewhere, anywhere, in anyone. I understood, viscerally and instantly, why men like to fuck so much. I couldn't feel a thing with my dick, but even so, I wanted to fuck everything in sight! It made a convenient resting place for my hand. It was fun to wag it around and strike "masculine" poses. I even found myself masturbating it, which felt good, actually. So much became clear at that moment. If only men could experience the equivalent with an artificial pussy, I suspect that there would be more harmony and less discord between the sexes.

When it's your turn to wield the strap-on, start with a toy longer than you think you'll need, since some extra length provides visual help in guiding it. Silicone "donuts," designed for use on the ends of vacuum tubes some men use to masturbate, are excellent accessories. They're not expensive and make a "bumper" at the base of the toy that effectively approximates the feel of a well-padded pubic bone and covers up any uncomfortable hardware that would otherwise dig in where it shouldn't. It makes it possible to sink completely into your partner's vaginal or anal anatomy and allows him or her to grind back on you in complete comfort. Here's how I load up my harness: a condom over the entire dildo (since I prefer both silicone lube and silicone toys), then the dildo in the harness, then the donut, then strapping on the entire contraption last. In general, harnessing up an eight-inch toy this way will leave you with six inches of usable penetration, which is about right for nearly everyone. Dildos designed only for anal play are generally smoother and thinner than those intended for vaginal use, though an experienced butt player can be amazingly accommodating. An added tip: If your partner's penis is truly too long for you, he can wear a donut himself to avoid hurting your cervix.

Some will find strap-on harnesses silly contraptions, more than a little weird, at first. When a woman gets over her giggles and puts one on, she often gets a rush of power and lust, which is very telling. Pair her with a partner who really likes penetration, and she'll soon conquer her initial inhibitions. The secret to fucking with a strap-on, beyond choosing one that fits properly, is to have a good mental picture of the interior terrain you're exploring with your numb toy and then to give yourself over to being active. Fuck your partner the way you like to be fucked or have seen others fuck. Learn to loosen your hips and wiggle the toy deeply inside. Get it all the way in, then gently roll around or move your hips only slightly. Your partner's response will tell you everything. Practice makes perfect. For couples exploring male-receptive anal

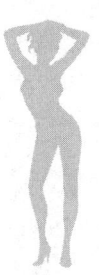

play, strap-on sex provides prostate stimulation and full-body contact as nothing else quite does.

Why would a man want to wear a strap-on? Some men are no longer able to get erections but would still like to fuck their partners in a familiar way. Some have already come for the evening, but their partner wants more. Strap-ons are useful in determining just how a woman likes to be fucked without the distraction of a throbbing hard-on. If you're playing power games, you can "deny" her your real cock and feed her an artificial one. With dildos, there's no worry about disease or pregnancy, and she can try out different "cocks" within a monogamous relationship. There are even harnesses with two holes, one above the other, designed so a man can place his penis through one hole, a dildo in the other, and penetrate a woman vaginally and anally at the same time. Depending on her position, his real cock can be in whichever orifice she prefers. This is much less complicated than trying to find that elusive extra dude!

We've already covered butt plugs in our chapter on anal play. To recap briefly, a butt plug is designed to fit snugly and comfortably into a person's anus and stay there. Some are worn during vaginal fucking by either the male or female partner, and some are designed for butt-only play. There is one new style, the Aneros, created expressly for men's hands-free prostate stimulation, and several of my male friends swear by it.

When it comes to toys engineered to simulate male anatomy, the choices are nearly as diverse. Jack-off sleeves, often made of cyberskin or super-stretchy silicone, come in all sorts of bright colors and funny shapes. There are also molded mouths, pussies, and/or butts of various porn performers. These are meant to give a man something new to masturbate with besides his hand, and they have a delicious, soft, smooth texture that many men find very exciting. They're easy to clean and portable. They can also be used as teaching aids to show a partner exactly how a vulva or butt should be stimulated, all while you're still dressed!

Many men like to play with cock rings or cock leashes. A cock ring, usually made of rubber, though some are made of metal, fits around a man's cock and balls, holding them snugly. When he's hard, the blood has a harder time flowing out, so cock rings can help a man maintain his erection. Before using a metal cock ring, have the clerk explain clearly how it works and how it goes on and off. If you're not comfortable asking that, you might want to stick with the rubber ones, which can, in event of an emergency, be cut off. A friend of mine used one on just his cock. I asked where he had found it, and he said it was an "O" ring he got at the auto shop for a dollar! Whatever works, I say! Cock leashes, which go around his whole package, are also fun to play with ("leading him by the balls" takes on a whole new meaning when it's literal), and the gentle tugging feels really good to a lot of men. If he likes it when you tug or hold his stuff with your hand, he's a good candidate for trying out a leash or a ball stretcher. Ball stretchers are little cuffs made of leather or cloth that are placed around the scrotum directly above the testicles, and close with snaps. Anywhere from one to four inches wide, they exert a steady, firm, hands-free pulling sensation that many men find delicious. Some men like to go out wearing their cock rings or ball stretchers under their clothes as part of foreplay, which is hot, I think.

Be aware that cock rings and other constricting devices carry certain risks. They work by restricting blood flow to the genitalia. Obviously, such practices require realistic time limits. Injuries ranging from broken capillaries to collapsed vesicles can result from overuse of con-

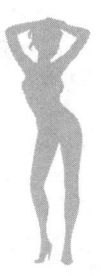

stricting toys. Once again, common sense dictates moderation. Don't wear anything around your cock that's uncomfortably tight or for longer than twenty minutes, even if it feels good at the time. Remember that sexual arousal dulls awareness of pain.

Some men and an increasing number of women have discovered the delights to be had by the application of suction to the genitals. Penis and pussy pumps, which use Lucite tubes connected to hand-operated or electrically driven vacuum devices, can create spectacular engorgement and enhanced sensitivity in erectile tissues of both genders. Intermittent mechanical suction can be a wonderful masturbatory aid, and the temporary swelling produced by such equipment can be both visually exciting and physically arousing by exposing more erotic surface to further stimulation. Contrary to some manufacturers' claims, such devices do not produce permanent enlargement of external organs and if used to excess can produce bruising and other unwanted side effects, so some caution is in order. Nonetheless, based on personal experience, I rate responsible vacuum play as a highly enjoyable supplement to other preliminaries prior to intercourse.

Beyond these basic pleasure enhancers lies a realm of more sophisticated and expensive high-tech toys you may wish to investigate when you're feeling both particularly adventurous and especially flush. One promising new form of toy play is electrostimulation, using low-powered transformers to deliver rhythmic electrical pulses to conductive cock rings, butt plugs, and dildos. As with so-called passive-exercise machines, the low-voltage current causes involuntary muscular contractions that mimic those produced by orgasm. Used in conjunction with more conventional forms of stimulation, electroplay can extend and enhance orgasmic response with impressive results. Obviously, there is danger whenever electricity is brought into contact with the human body. No electrical device should ever be used above the waist, given the risk of triggering cardiac arrhythmias (the heart is itself, after all, an electrical pump), and inadvertent shocks at the wrong moment are no fun whatsoever. With any electrical toy, follow the instructions carefully, proceed with caution, and desist at the first sign of discomfort.

It was inevitable from the creation of the first dildo that somebody would try to engineer a means of making one function like a real penis without the need for a human life-support system. Automated fucking machines date from the Victorian era but only recently have they come into their own. It's now possible to purchase, at significant expense, piston-driven, motorized fuck toys capable of producing anything from a slow, shallow stroke to a pounding Brahma bull ride. Shafts can be adjusted for angle and depth of penetration, and either the recipient or a partner can control speed of operation. Attachments can be exchanged for different sizes and shapes. I have some experience with these gadgets and find them terrific fun. It's like having an extra guy available when you want him who has no ego to worry about, doesn't need a cigarette afterward, and never asks you your sign. These tireless, ever-patient mechanical slaves are worth the heavy chunk of change they cost for those who can afford them.

Out of the Closet and into Your Bed

How do you bring up the subject of sex toys with a partner? With tact and firmness. When it comes to sharing pleasure, there's nothing two adults shouldn't be able to discuss. Keep in mind that the need or desire for a toy is not a negative comment on the abilities of your lover. You may feel guilty for needing the extra stimulation of a vi-

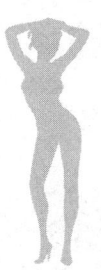

brator in order to come. Your partner may feel hurt over not being "enough" for you. Don't waste time and feelings on such notions. Your individual, orgasmic wiring is what it is, and you need what you need to get off. There's no right or wrong here, only what's true.

Likewise, you needn't feel pressured to perform "like a porn star" if your partner brings home a toy, when all he wants to do is see you have more pleasure. If your or your partner's reaction to the subject of toys is negative, look inside for what the real issues might be. If your sexual communication isn't what it should be, bringing home a toy won't change that, and communication needs to precede the introduction of a potentially threatening new element to your lovemaking. Instead of feeling less than adequate because your lover needs a buzz in order to get over the edge, find ways to help her. Hold her breasts, work the dildo, cuddle her, whisper naughty things in her ear, or masturbate beside her. Find a way for pleasure to bring you closer, not push you apart.

Generally, the desire for toys is a positive one, meaning that the person is ready and willing to explore different ways to share pleasure, ready to expand an already happy sex life into new territories. Many couples have a toy box that sits always ready just within reach or a locking toy drawer next to the bed. Locking is a good idea, since you never know who may be "just looking around" your bedroom!

Sex toys can get very specific, and it's fun to experiment until you find the perfect toy for what you need. Think creatively and pragmatically. A toy designed for butt use won't be so good for vaginal penetration. The little vibrator may be fun for teasing, but the Big Gun might be needed for the final orgasm. On some days, you may want the bigger dildo; on others, the bent one or the fat one or the skinny one. On a greedy day, a butt can be very expandable. On another occasion, it's the skinny toy or none at all. The toys that I use almost every time are my Hitachi and my favorite butt plug, with the others "filling in" as needed.

The most important thing to remember is that a sex toy serves to enhance a satisfying, functional sexual relationship, not supplant it. No mechanical artifact can take the place of real emotional intimacy. As long as this principle forms the context in which toys are used, they offer opportunities to increase enjoyment without overwhelming human contact.

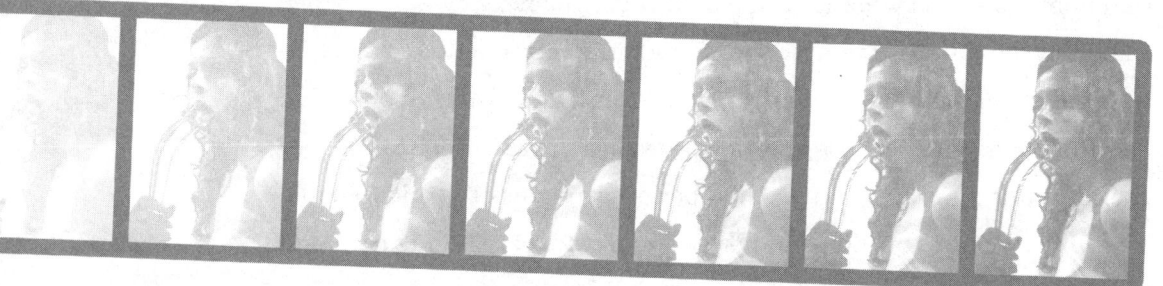

TIPS FOR TOYS

1 • *Have no fear.* They're inanimate objects with no minds of their own and can do only what you make them do.

2 • *Let your body lead you.* If it feels good, it's a good toy; if not, not.

3 • *Try to see your partner's desire for toys positively.* It means he or she is interested in better sex with you, which is the whole idea.

4 • *Be a sensible shopper.* Before purchasing the shiny, expensive widget, really look it over. Have the store clerk get out a demonstrator and turn it on so you can evaluate how well it will work for you.

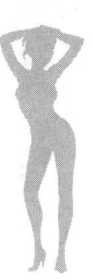

5 • *Get over your resistance to toys.* A vibrator can mean the difference between a lukewarm partner and a hot one.

6 • *Bring your partner along for the shopping trip.* You might find out something new and useful.

7 • *Give a new toy a couple of chances before abandoning it as a bad purchase.* Some take a bit of practice to master.

8 • *When you find something that works for you, get an extra and keep it handy.* You're likely to wear out the first one sooner than you think.

TOY TRAPS

1 • *Don't spring a new toy on your partner right before playing.* Give him or her a chance to check it out first in a more neutral setting.

2 • *Just because it caught your eye in the store doesn't mean your partner will go for it.* Show some common sense. That huge, porn-stud silicone cock might just end up as a handy-dandy home defense device, and you'll be out lots of money.

3 • *Don't frantically thrust and jab a toy into any orifice.* Instead, feel your way around inside and be guided by the sounds of pleasure or discomfort.

4 • *Avoid using the vibrator as a labor-saving device.* Don't just plant it on your partner's clit and grind away until you both get bored and annoyed. Follow the lead of her signals, using more pressure or less, turning the speed up or down, etc. Stay in touch.

5 • *Never neglect toy hygiene.* They need thorough cleaning after each use.

6 • *With any electrical or mechanical toy, do not fail to read the instructions thoroughly.* Know how they work before trying them with a partner.

7 • *Never belittle a partner for needing a mechanical assist.* You'll only be exhibiting your own insecurities.

8 • *Don't knock a toy until you've tried it.* Some rather unlikely-looking items turn out to have great potential. Use your imagination when visualizing how they might operate.

Chapter 12

SWINGING:
STRANGERS AT THE PARTY

winging can be loosely defined as any kind of organized recreational sex involving more than one couple. Though not as visible a presence on the pop-culture radar as it was thirty years ago, it's actually more popular than ever. Hundreds of thousands of practitioners from coast to coast gather regularly for local, regional, and national conventions as well as countless parties on Friday and Saturday nights in their hometowns. With various adaptations to changes in the larger society, swinging seems to be enjoying something of a renaissance among a younger generation of participants. The big Saturday-night theme dance at the last national Alternative Lifestyles convention I attended drew three thousand couples who had the time of their lives. Bear in mind that for every couple who attends the larger events, a hundred more dream of doing so.

You can't tell swingers by looking; you may even live next door to some, as they're understandably discreet. Swinging is mainly a development of Western cultures that have well-defined middle and upper classes. It's an activity requiring a fair amount of leisure time and disposable income as well as a liberated attitude toward sexuality in general and women's sexuality in particular. I've long said that swinging is a parallel universe, where people look like you and me but where the accepted rules and social boundaries regarding sexual intimacy have been shifted by mutual agreement. Contemporary swinging has little in common with the seventies'-era "key parties" or "wife-swapping parties" depicted by Gay Talese in his daring-for-its-time book *Thy Neighbor's Wife,* though it did grow out of the new thinking about sex, gender, and culture that burst forth into public consciousness during that decade.

At its best, swinging is not cheating, predatory, an expression of low self-esteem, a cop-out to avoid intimacy, inherently dangerous, mentally unbalanced, or unethical. It is an expression of a sexual orientation, akin to being gay or monogamous. Those so inclined accept their fantasies and desires and seek to act them out in healthy ways with others of like mind. This is not to suggest that swinging is just a variant of ordinary social or sexual behavior or that those who engage in it are unexceptional. Simply admitting that they like to engage in sex with other people while their partners are present sets swingers apart from the majority. For the most part, however, the sex itself is "regular": simple nudity, hugging, kissing, sucking, and fucking, spiced with exhibitionism, voyeurism, partner swapping, and group sex.

Swinging involves social as well as sexual intercourse. Many couples

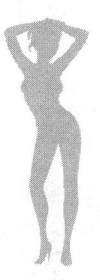

form strong and long-lasting friendships. They get together for nonsexual events such as picnics with all the kids or going to the movies. Observing a group of swingers out in public, it's hard not to be struck by how close they appear to be, how relaxed and at ease the men and women are with one another. They've discovered for themselves how refreshing and liberating it is to put aside doctrinal notions of "normal" sexual behavior and forge their own, custom-built community of fellow travelers. In this way swinging is like any other affinity group, secular or religious. The men are relaxed because they no longer have to compete with one another for access to women or wonder in silence if a potential partner shares their interest. The women are happy to be the center of attention and desire and to feel fully appreciated (as opposed to shamed) for their robust interest in all things sexual. They also know that the female partners in swinging couples make all decisions involving partner choice and activities pursued. For those so inclined, swinging is the perfect way to balance impulses we've been told are antithetical: romance and mating versus freewheeling sexual activity with multiple partners.

Swinging tends to amplify the underlying strengths and weaknesses of relationships and, as such, is no way for couples in trouble to "fix" things. If a couple is solid and shares the inclination fully, swinging can be a wonderful addition to an already healthy and satisfying sex life. If there are cracks or stresses within a marriage, swinging will only serve to bring them to the surface. Keeping in mind that no outside force can break up a happy marriage, swinging poses no threat to a solid union. But a couple's house must be in order before attempting anything so radical as inviting others into the bedroom. A happy swinging couple and a happy committed couple are one and the same.

Who Are They, Anyway?

In most people's lives there is a period of sexual experimentation and dating followed by mating, marriage, and monogamy. Thereafter, they're happy to keep any sexual exploration within the boundaries of the dyad. Swingers, however, want to have their cake (a committed relationship) and eat it, too (have sexy fun with others). Along the continuum of relationship styles, swinging falls between monogamy and polyamory. A swinger's romantic ties are reserved for his or her primary partner. He or she may have strong friendships with other swingers, some warmer and closer than others, but no outside romantic attachments are permitted or desired. Unlike polyamory, group living or group marriage is not on the agenda for swingers, though group vacations are common.

Swingers hail from all walks of life, exhibiting a striking diversity in age, race, ethnicity, and religious and political affiliations. There are working-class swingers, of course, but they tend to play close to home with friends and don't often make it to the big conventions because of budget constraints. Rich people can be swingers, too, but they tend to avoid public gatherings for obvious reasons. Most of the swingers you'll meet are solidly middle class. They are often surprisingly conventional, even conservative, in all but their sexual activities. Many are dedicated, involved parents. I've seen more than one couple leave a party at three in the morning to be home in time to take their kids to Sunday school.

People find their way to the swinging world from many different starting points, but all report a sense of feeling at home as soon as they take the leap by attending a party or other swinger event, even if they hang back from direct participation at first. I was destined to be a

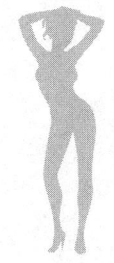

swinger by the time I understood that I was bisexual, even though I didn't yet know the term. Unlike many, I never wanted, or offered, monogamy. I wanted a life where I could be open about myself and find others who shared my vision. We often don't recognize how oppressive the prevailing rules are until we depart from them, even if for only one evening, so it was a revelation to discover that many others shared my inclinations. Even if I hadn't been so exhibitionistic as to become a sex performer, I'd still be a swinger. In that sense, I'm an anomaly in the swinging world also, as I would have sought it out whether I had a steady partner or not.

While being far from scientific, I've observed that the two most common types of swingers are high school or college sweethearts who have grown together and found this world together and those in happy second marriages, each person having been previously married to sexually incompatible partners before breaking away to find happiness on his or her own terms. Some people do marry and then discover this aspect of their sexuality. Some marriages can grow to accommodate such discoveries, but most, in the end, cannot, since swinging and monogamy are incompatible relationship preferences. Swingers are people who want to be honest and open about their sexuality, to make their peace with it, and to live the dream. Neither sullen fidelity nor sweaty-palmed adultery will do as a substitute.

Why Do They Act Like That?

For a certain type of person, swinging is the best way to satisfy a deep longing for variety with none of the pitfalls of the single-and-dating scene, which, by definition, excludes mated people. Some are naturally free of jealousy; others, like me, have rid themselves of this poisonous emotion in order to live the life they want. In a swing environment the normal rules governing body boundaries and permissible behavior are turned inside out. If you're new to the scene, you'll find swingers eager to share their experiences: how they started, how they've handled relationship issues, what they've done to overcome their inhibitions and insecurities, and other practical details of living an "alternative lifestyle."

The impetus to swing is often powered by a woman's bisexuality or exhibitionism. Most women in the swing world are bisexual or at least "bi-curious." Their husbands want them to be happy and to share in the fun themselves by way of voyeurism. Some couples have gone to the limit of what sexual experimentation they can do with each other, including sharing fantasies of other partners and, finding that thought sexy rather than scary, feel ready to take the step of including another person for real.

As often as swinging provides opportunities for a woman to find pussy and dance naked in a crowd, it also offers a loving wife the chance to fulfill a husband's fantasy. Whatever motivates the initial urge to experiment, it's safe to say that the reality of swinging invariably comes as a surprise. Husbands and wives may have very different and sometimes conflicting visions of what will actually occur. He may picture himself attacked by a bevy of eager, horny women and dragged to a corner to meet his happy fate. She may fear she'll be set upon by a bunch of troglodytes and dragged to a corner to meet a fate worse than death. What they can't know until they encounter it firsthand is that the social contract at a swing party makes either outcome unlikely. Women are in charge of the sexual negotiations, and a level of decorum somewhat reminiscent of that of a high-school prom (though with less clothing) generally prevails. Once in attendance at the much discussed,

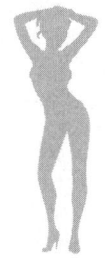

long-awaited party, the woman finds that she's perfectly safe among people who are charming and flirty, and the man soon learns that he must make friends first in order to recruit partners for his imaginary bacchanal. Hours later, she's having the time of her life, while he can't wait to get out of there. I've seen such couples work through their issues and continue happily in the lifestyle, while others crash and burn over their differing experiences and expectations. If you haven't already surmised so on your own, let me say in all honesty that swinging is not for everybody.

Breaking the Ice, Not the Rules

In some important respects, swinging is a woman's paradise. Among swingers, a woman with a powerful sex drive and a robust appetite is respected, revered, desired, and emulated instead of reviled, pitied, scorned, and ostracized. Women dominate swinging culture, and don't let anyone tell you otherwise. If she doesn't say "yes," sex doesn't happen. Unlike the "real" world, in the alternative universe of swinging, a woman can have as much or as little attention as she wants with no one thinking less of her. Things that can get a woman into trouble in public—flashing her butt or boobs, rubbing the crotch of a hot guy, kissing her girlfriend—are welcomed at a swing party. Things that can get a man beaten up by an irate husband—complimenting another woman's body, casually offering her some oral sex—are regarded as polite overtures among swingers.

By attending a swing party, you signal that you're interested in sex and at the very least are willing to talk about it. You can ask a person nearly anything in a respectful manner without risk of offense. Anyone can refuse any request, and refusals must be accepted without argument. It's such a relief to be in a place where you can talk freely about sexual matters without disapproval from others that many otherwise monogamous couples go to parties just to dance, flirt, show off, and converse with sexually liberated adults. Over the years, I've seen countless women blossom from shy creatures hiding behind their husband's protective arms to confident party starters and cheerleaders for other newcomers.

Every group needs its initiators. Exhibitionist that I am, I'm usually the first one naked, pulling in a willing woman for a hot show to get the ball rolling. This certainly enhances my popularity, but it is by no means expected of every woman in attendance. The best way to behave at a party is honestly. If you're new to the scene, don't pretend you're not. At first, a new couple will generate a lot of interest and not a few invitations to join others in the play areas. While a simple, polite "No, thank you" should be sufficient, it can help to add: "We're new to all of this and still finding our way." Everyone was new once, and they'll understand. Often, there will be a designated "care couple," there to ensure that newcomers aren't overwhelmed and unable to mingle. As your explorations expand, you'll find you like some people more than others, or one member of a couple better than the other. You'll find different couples odious and overbearing, standoffish and remote, quiet and shy, warm and accessible, attractive or not. In that way, too, swinging is rather like high school but with the sex out in the open. If you stick around the scene long enough, you'll find people with whom you click and make lifelong friends.

Safer-sex precautions are a must when you first get into swinging. Condoms for intercourse are standard for beginners, though oral sex is usually bareback with either gender. Don't be shocked to see long-term swinging friends dispense with condoms. People who swing rarely

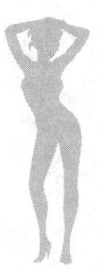

play outside the community and tend to form close affinity groups within it. Once trust is established, they often do away with barrier protections. It's also become increasingly common for regular play partners to get tested for STDs, sharing the results before sharing bodily fluids. Swingers think of themselves as a community of friends, and friends don't put one another at risk. This is one reason why, despite the dire predictions of twenty years ago, swinging culture neither collapsed with the onset of HIV nor became a breeding ground for infection. Another safety factor in both porn and swinging is the standard practice of external ejaculation. Swinging men rarely ejaculate internally with anyone other than a primary partner. Given the emphasis on variety, it's also common for swinging men to fuck multiple women at a party without ejaculating once.

I recommend seeking your own comfort level with other couples on a case-by-case basis. When in doubt, err on the side of safety. If you need to use condoms in order to relax enough to play, do so. In group-sex situations, be aware that some men can't perform with condoms very well, so early encounters may go no further than mutual masturbation or a blow job. That's not a bad way to get to know a potential playmate before moving on to more intimate forms of contact.

Proceed with Caution

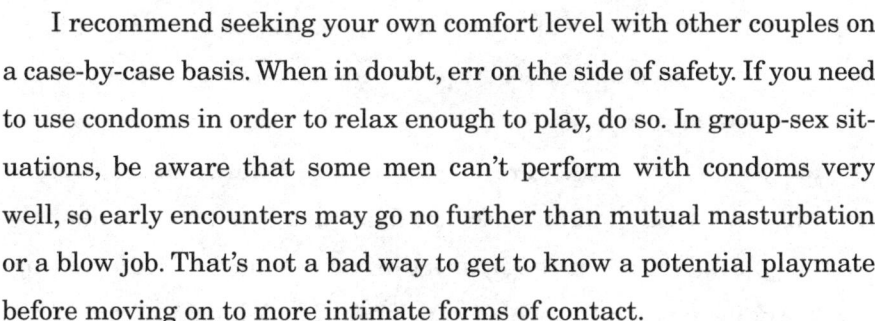

There is a wealth of information regarding swinging, both in print and online, and you should investigate all you can before taking any bold initiatives. Talk it all out. Share fully and honestly what you like about the idea of swinging and what causes you concern. If you can't address your reservations in private, you're unlikely to resolve them happily in public. What attracts you to the idea of swinging? How do you feel about your partner touching someone else in a sexual manner? How does your partner feel about you touching someone else in a sexual manner? What will you do if discord arises? Your reasons are always valid if they proceed from real feeling, but you must own them. Until you can have this conversation with complete candor and generosity, you're not ready to leave home.

No matter how much homework you've done, no matter how much the idea excites you, no matter how often you've talked it over with your partner, neither of you can know for sure how you'll actually feel and respond to your first swing event. Finally acting out a long-held fantasy can be pretty overwhelming, especially when it involves breaking the fourth wall between a couple and potential lovers. To do so goes against all that we've been told is right, that society says is healthy and moral. Confronting this reality can unearth insecurities you didn't know you had, so be prepared to be surprised at your own reaction to what you see, hear, and experience.

You and your partner are a team. If the team's not functioning smoothly, the team shouldn't take the field. As a team, you should have your playbook laid out in detail, including your behavior limits and signals to indicate when they've been reached. Though both of you might be shy when you first get to a party, one of you might warm up much faster and be ready for the starting gun before the other. Decide ahead of time that you'll stick close by and check in with each other frequently. Remember I said that total sex is generous? That generosity extends to yourself as well as to others. This is not the time to go along to get along. If it turns out that one of you is less comfortable with a prospective encounter than the other, those reservations should be respected. If you're meant for this kind of recreation, there will be other opportunities.

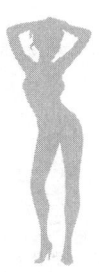

Don't drink to compensate for your nervousness. One is fine; more than that is a sure sign of discomfort that shouldn't be ignored. As with any form of sexual experimentation, if you need to be drunk or high to move past your inhibitions, go home and save yourself the humiliation of barfing on someone or passing out in a corner. That's the part of high school you don't need to relive. If you find yourself in a sexual situation that doesn't feel right and have to pull back, you can do so smoothly by using a coded signal you and your primary partner have chosen in advance. "Oh my God, the dog!" works well. Your partner will know that means "I need to go NOW" and must honor your request by disengaging politely from what he or she is doing so you can leave together. Smile on the way out and save all discussions for the car. Open bickering is considered one of the worst social gaffes among swingers.

There are several in-between stages a couple can pass through as they map out their comfort zone. If the woman wants to experiment with exhibitionism, she can request a ten-handed full-body massage but declare her pussy off-limits. She'll get five takers pronto. Parallel play, so-called "soft swinging," combines exhibitionism and voyeurism without crossing the line into partner swapping. Two couples can make love on adjoining beds within sight of each other but have no cross-couple contact. This look-but-don't-touch approach is a great intermediate step. The next move often involves the two women playing while their partners watch, with the understanding that each man will touch only his own companion. From there, if you've found the right company, exchanges of oral sex are often next on the agenda, with intercourse still reserved for the original couples.

Many couples never go beyond these titillations to actual partner exchange. Others are destined to expand their horizons as far as possible. I know one man who loves to see his wife take on as many men as she can in one evening. He stays by her and hands out the condoms but doesn't fuck her until they get home. She's the exhibitionist and he's the voyeur, which makes for easy compatibility in public circumstances. It's common for a couple to have all sorts of fun at a party, but, no matter how many partners each one may have had, he saves his last orgasm for her, signaling the end of the evening. As a girlfriend of mine put it, "Once I've had my home cock, I'm done for the night!"

There are those who prefer to stay together at all times, both as a mutual turn-on and to provide a sense of comfort and security. This is a good way to go while any residual jealousy or insecurity issues are worked out. By playing together, each partner knows exactly what happened, that safer-sex techniques were used, and that no emotional or behavioral boundaries were crossed.

Others play a bit separately but prefer to remain within visual proximity. Then there are those who say, "Just don't leave the house, sweetheart!" At the far, rather rarified, end of the spectrum are couples like me and my husband, who are comfortable playing separately when one or the other is out of town, then telling each other the juicy details later. I've always been this way. My particular vision of liberated sexuality of this type is not a goal to be achieved but a preference to be discovered, if it's there. The crucial element for fun, safe, emotionally comfortable swinging is reaching a mutually satisfactory compromise between your desires and your boundaries. How other couples handle their particular situations is not to be copied, but it is to be discussed, the better for you and your partner to find what's best for you. Swinging is a 100 percent made-to-order activity.

It's important that all four members of any two couples establish their compatibility before any further activity is negotiated. If both of you like her but hate him, it's no good, and vice versa. For me, it's less

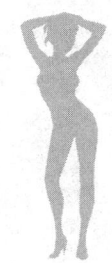

about physical attractiveness and more about personal connection. I'm not dating him or having his baby, so how hunky (or not) he may be isn't my primary concern. I often make my choices, at least in part, based on how people interact as couples. Do they seem happy together, in sync with each other, warm and friendly? If so, they may get a second look, whereas a more conventionally attractive pair who come off as cool but superficial may get a pass. The critical point here is that all decisions must be unanimous. For example, we know one supernice couple we both enjoy socially. She's gorgeous and he's . . . well . . . not. He's nice, don't get me wrong, but conventionally handsome he ain't (though he assures us he's a love god in private, and I don't doubt him). I was willing to play with them, since I liked them both and wanted to see my husband with her, but my husband wasn't interested in seeing him with me, no matter how hot he was for her, so it just hasn't happened. All vetoes carry equal weight.

What to Bring to a Sex Party

The most important things to bring to a sex party are a good attitude and good manners. You're in a new social milieu, and you'll make your best impression by not trying to impress. The next most important items on the list are warm, comfy clothes to wear home. That killer mini dress with the towering high heels that you wore to wow everyone are so not what you want to put on in the wee hours after a rockin' good time. Bring sweats, hoodies, sneakers, and, at the very least, fuzzy slippers and a big warm coat, so you can bundle up and be comfy on the way home from your big night. You'll need the big coat, anyway, to cover yourself up from the car to the party. Your "gym bag" should also contain hair ties, a hairbrush, a travel robe, your favorite condoms, lube, latex gloves, toys (dildos, vibrators, leashes, paddles, etc.), baby wipes, and any special snacks you think you might want. The party hosts will have a refreshment table and they often provide safer-sex supplies, but if you can't eat the usual chips, dip, and cookies, make sure you have fuel for the activities you hope to enjoy, since nothing ruins a good time more than hunger pangs. Trust me, you'll work up an appetite!

Many swing parties are built around a theme: Leather and Lingerie, School Girls and Lettermen, Boxer-Short Brigade, No-Panty Party, Rock 'n' Roll, Valentine Vixens, Halloween Hump, Santa and His Elves, Pole Dance Contest, etc. Respect the hosts by dressing accordingly. The women tend to be more stylish than the guys, and the early stages of a party are often taken up with the women admiring one another's outfits while the men admire the women. Dress up enough to feel special but not self-conscious. All body types are welcome at swing parties, but I'd be lying if I didn't say that mainstream notions of attractiveness prevail. This is where good grooming, dress, and personal hygiene can be very helpful. Swingers respect the effort in making the most of what nature gave you.

Parties held at hotels are more circumspect than those at private homes. When the event is booked in a ballroom, sexy but not nude is the rule. Nipples, butts, and genitals must be covered at all times, which makes flirting and showing off an entertaining challenge. People hook up and retire to the rooms upstairs for more intimate purposes. Some encounters are spontaneous, and some dates are planned in advance. For bigger gatherings, a whole floor of suites can be rented by the group, which makes for some lively and at times faintly farcical running in and out of rooms. At events in private homes, there is often a room set aside for nonsexual activity to give the shy folks a place of

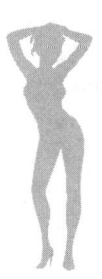

retreat, but the rules are a lot looser, with nudity and sex permitted everywhere else. A donation box is often used to offset the costs of hosting: extra laundry, food and beverages, safer-sex supplies, etc. Give what you can.

Some cities have established swing clubs, either "on premise" or "off premise." At an on-premise club, you can meet another couple and play with them on the spot. Membership is usually required, and, as in most swing venues, single men are not permitted (I know it sucks, but ill-mannered men have ruined it for the rest). If you're already members in good standing of a club and can vouch for a single male friend and take responsibility for him, some clubs will stretch that rule, as some women prefer to play with multiple male partners. At an off-premise club, you meet and negotiate, then leave the club in order to play, usually in a nearby hotel room you've already rented. As a rule, avoid taking people you've just met back to your place. While I've had very few unpleasant, much less threatening, experiences in many years of swinging, a certain wariness toward strangers is just common sense.

Making Sure You're Invited Back

The most important way to make sure you're not eighty-sixed from a party or permanently struck from the guest list is to leave the drama at home. If there are issues between the two of you, keep them to yourselves or stay home and deal with them. Nothing is more off-putting to potential playmates than a visibly unhappy couple. They ruin the mood for everyone else. If you simply can't control yourselves, leave quietly after thanking your hosts. Treat each other well in front of others. We all hate it when one partner really wants to be in the swinging environment while the other is clearly uncomfortable but too insecure to admit it. Pressuring your partner to do anything sexual that he or she resists is also bad form. If your partner isn't eagerly grabbing for the other person's crotch, don't push. If your swinging "dial" is turned to ten while your S.O.'s is at four, more negotiation is needed. Take it outside, and when you do, don't forget to cover up completely before leaving the house. Don't be naked anywhere the host couple says is a no-go area. Your hosts' neighbors may not be swing friendly. Don't park where it's forbidden, and be quiet going to and from the house.

No Regrets

The day after a swinging experience, both you and your partner should feel happy and secure. The love you have for him or her should be deepened and that love returned in kind. Feelings of contentment, joy, gratitude, and satisfaction are evidence that a good time was had by all. How often you engage in this extracurricular activity is a matter of individual choice. One couple I know, together now thirty years, swung five nights a week for more than a decade, hosted events regularly, and were the life of any party. Once a month is more their speed now. Others are happy with twice a year, as a special treat. Swinging

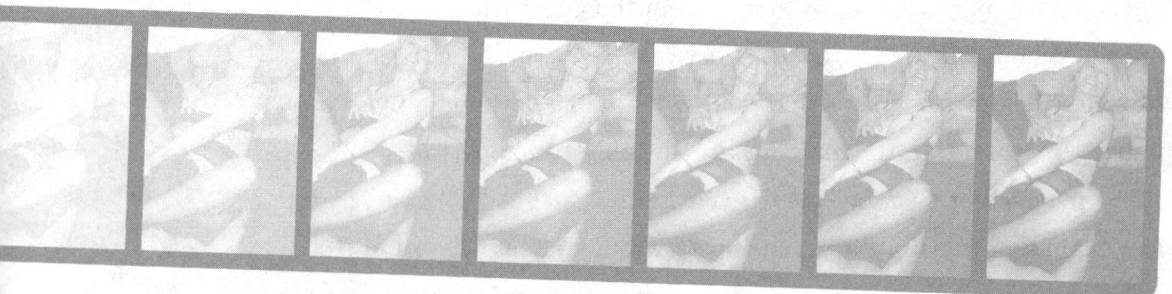

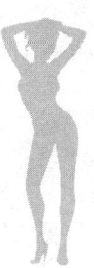

should only serve to solidify and protect a couple's commitment to each other. It may turn out to be an experimental phase that only validates your choice of a life mate. You may try swinging and grow out of it, and in later years recall your wilder days with fondness—a perfectly desirable outcome.

SWINGING FOR THE BLEACHERS

1 • *Do your homework about this community before getting started.* You wouldn't travel overseas without reading a guidebook. Don't tackle the wilds of swinging without a road map.

2 • *Keep an open mind.* You'll find out things about yourself or your partner that will surprise you. You may discover new ways of turning you both on . . . and off.

3 • *Be prepared to expand your definition of a good time.* You may find you like to watch more than you expected.

4 • *Plan ahead for any contingency.* Have what you need at the time you need it. You shouldn't have to worry about forgetting your contact lens case.

5 • *Have your ID and some cash with you, but leave other valuables at home.*

6 • *Mingle freely with the crowd.* You might make wonderful new friends, even if there's no physical interaction.

7 • *It's okay to be shy or unsure of yourselves.* Every couple was new once, so someone will help you out. Just remember to pay it forward when you're the veterans.

8 • *Happy people are attractive.* Decide in advance to make it a hot date together, regardless of what does or does not happen with others.

GROUP GRIPES

1 • *Manners matter, so don't be rude to each other or anybody else.* If others fail to observe this rule, report it to your hosts.

2 • *Don't come on too strong to people you don't know.* Flirting is fine, but touching without permission is verboten. Ask the person you're interested in, not his or her partner.

3 • *Don't let any emotional meltdown trickle over onto others.* If you can't keep it together, call it a night.

4 • *Don't mistreat your partner in front of others (or anywhere else),* lest you become The Couple Nobody Wants. Even worse, your partner will be The Spouse Everyone Pities.

5 • *Another person's limits and boundaries are to be respected. No* means "no," and the person doesn't have to explain or say it more than once.

6 • *Don't endanger the hosts' security by raucous behavior.* They have to live there between parties.

7 • *Keep your less flattering judgments of others to yourself.* You never know who might be listening.

8 • *Watching is fine, but do not join in any others' activities without being invited.* You want your space respected; so do they.

Chapter 13

THREE-WAY SEX:
TWO GIRLS AND A GUY—
MORE FUN THAN IT SOUNDS

Much like performing sex for an audience, being with a man and a woman at the same time is as natural to me as breathing and just as vital. In response to the FAQ of whether I prefer men or women, I always say I'll take one of each. The playdate of choice for me and my husband is another woman. Between the jealousy-driven love-triangle dramas of popular entertainment and the fantasy fluff of porn mini orgies lies an actual terrain rich in possibilities for love, intimacy, adventure, and unexpected friendships. Of all group-sex scenarios, the boy-girl-girl three-way is not only the most popular but also the most likely. To my delight (and the horror of others), on any given night thousands of couples play happily with a special girlfriend, or two gal pals bring home a lucky guy to share.

As many a man who bought into the pornographic cliché version of such situations has discovered upon finding himself outnumbered in bed, the agenda is less apt to be all about him and what he wants than it is about them and what they want. If you're wired this way, threesomes offer a most unusual opportunity for female bonding, even if the women are not bisexual. While cultural taboos require men to be on their guard around each other, thus making a two-man/one-woman party especially tricky, women are permitted close same-sex friendships and casual physical affection. Those women who can add sex to the mix enjoy unique social advantages. A woman who can experience other women as lovers or allies rather than as rivals in her relations with men can find an inexhaustible source of pleasure and support among like-minded coconspirators.

Lest I be accused of painting too rosy a portrait, there are some caveats that come with the endorsement: Threesomes, however transient, are still relationships, which are freighted with all the usual perils of manipulation, dishonesty, selfishness, and unwanted discoveries that attend any intimate embrace. Not all the risks of opening the bedroom door to a third party are imaginary. Threesomes strengthen my marriage today, but both my husband and I agree that they played a largely destructive role in our respective first marriages. Therefore, let us go bravely but cautiously along this path.

No matter who broaches the initial idea, the motivation to pursue a threesome must grow equally from all parties, whether they be confident friends or a secure, fulfilled primary couple and a trusted outsider. It's not enough for the gang to share a hot fantasy with one another, though that's surely a prerequisite to making it real one day. It's not enough for them to declare their wish to do so, though that discussion (always ongoing) is essential to success. A threesome will only live up

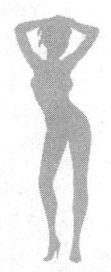

to expectations if all three parties bring the benefits of happy, satisfying sex lives of their own to the experience. Threesomes are like dessert that way: They're only good as part of an otherwise healthy diet. I've seen many failing couples try to sustain themselves on the borrowed sexual energy of outsiders only to be consumed from within by the emptiness they felt when alone with each other.

While spontaneous threesomes do occasionally erupt among singles, more commonly an established couple forms the base of the triad. What begins as a shared notion between the members eventually evolves into the active pursuit of a third participant. That evolution can be quite lengthy, with much discussion of what might or might not happen. Some couples entertain themselves with the threesome fantasy for many years before giving it a go. There's no reason to force the issue. Until you feel absolute confidence in your generosity toward each other, hold off. You and your primary partner are a team, and the team must function smoothly before adding to the line-up. Then there's still the problem of finding a compatible third. It's better to wait for the right person and situation to come along than to rush into something because you fear the opportunity might not present itself again. If you're not ready yet but your most likely third partner is moving to Italy next month, don't race to fit her into your social calendar. Instead, bid her a fond farewell and add her to your fantasy folder. Your mutual attraction to her is an important step toward the real thing later on. You and your partner may experience sexual attraction to many women before you bed one for real, and that's as it should be.

Use that little "zing" you got from reckless eyeballing at the mall to add heat to your time alone together. Discuss how it feels to see each other actually aroused by someone else. No fibbing. If jealousy is a deal breaker, it's less embarrassing to admit it in private than it will be in front of an audience. Learn to flirt as a team. It's a fun new way to bond with your mate and good practice for that first, butterflies-in-the-stomach, party-for-three dinner date. You'll be awkward the first few times you try out your act in public, but if threesomes are your thing, you'll eventually learn to play off each other like expert doubles players on a tennis court.

If your "team" consists of two female friends out for a hot time, the fishing will be easier, since men usually aren't difficult to entice with the help of a gal pal. "My girlfriend and I want to bring you home and play naked together" will usually do the trick, though you may be surprised by how many men flee in terror at the prospect of getting something of which they've dreamed their whole lives. Those who consent will generally prove very compliant with any rules you choose. But don't expect your relationship with your friend to be completely unaffected by the experience. You may not have as much at stake as you would with a mate, but close female companions have been known to fall out over guys neither one has ever fucked, much less a man they've shared. Here again, have your priorities straight before you commit: If one of you is just looking for fun and the other is hoping to snare a more permanent situation with the promise of unconventional pleasures, somebody's going to end up feeling used.

Writing Your Own Rules

If and when you're ready to move from talk to action, I can confidently assure you that when it finally happens the actual sexual encounter will not play out exactly as you expect. Still, it helps to go in with a plan of sorts. This kind of game needs rules. When I talk about

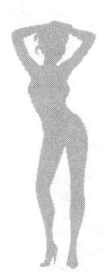

rules, I mean physical boundaries, such as who gets to touch whom and how, emotional protocols concerning displays of affection, and the diplomatic graces that keep the party frictionless. The only votes that count are those of the couple and their lover. Don't try to replicate how it looks in porn, which is all fantasy, or concern yourself with how others make it work, which is all conjecture. What are your fears? What are your hopes, fantasies, and desires? After you get past the teasing-and-flirting phase, you'll need to negotiate boundaries so that you all feel safe enough to really let go. Far from stripping your three-way of some imaginary spontaneity, you'll come to understand that a brief exchange of serious, grown-up talk beforehand liberates you to enjoy the transcendent fusion you came together to find. Once the party's under way and all involved see how they interact in practice, the rules can and will shift, sometimes dramatically and frequently in the direction of more openness. A player who feared seeing his or her partner kiss the guest may decide it would be hot to watch after all. But knowing in advance that specific limits will be observed is exactly what enables that kind relaxation. The safer the couple and lover feel as an entity, the more they'll enjoy their time together.

Here are some rules that I've seen work: Only the primary couple has intercourse, with the guest woman offering oral sex, petting, visual stimulation, and a very helpful extra pair of hands. The two women make love, with the man having contact exclusively with his S.O. The two women aren't bisexual, and thus keep him the focus at all times. He can't kiss the guest, but he can fuck her. He can kiss her and perform oral sex, and some friendly canoodling is okay, but hot and heavy romantic necking is reserved for his primary partner. The guest can stay for dinner but can't spend the night. The possible variations in the rule book are endless, and as long as they're honest and honestly agreed to, whatever necessary amendments can be made without upsetting the fundamentals of the agreement.

Having had so many threesomes, I know they're not always trouble-free, even if everything seems fine at the outset. Thought should be given to handling unexpected, and unwelcome, meltdowns. The proceedings can be going along just fine when something is triggered in one of the players, changing the mood instantly. The person with the sudden problem will likely be surprised and mortified, unwilling to express his or her feelings and possibly ruin things for the others. Such a problem needs to be addressed, however, since it will come out one way or another.

If the guest is the one who abruptly goes stiff and cold, stop to check in with her. It may turn out to be a fleeting hesitation, or she may need to excuse herself and go home. If you care for her and want to keep options open for the future, be gracious as you help her dress and show her to her car. It's a good sign if, should the party "dehappinate," the core couple is perfectly happy to continue alone.

Should one of the primary partners hit the wall, the same considerations apply. Don't push on and hope to straighten it all out later. No one deserves to hear a fight break out as she's leaving. If the issue is an internal one the couple needs to deal with privately, the guest should either make a graceful exit or, if she's a very good friend, stay and offer support. If nothing less than a full-engine shutdown is unavoidable, be sure to contact your third the next day to let her know everything's all right and to thank her for her understanding. Doubts and reservations can often be resolved in the cool light of day, and you might be pleasantly surprised at how easily you can pick up where you left off. If you do, you may all feel much closer after sharing something real.

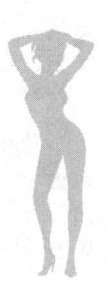

Respecting Masculine Insecurities

While the two-women-just-for-me fantasy is a staple for many men, when faced with the daunting prospect of actually "satisfying" both, any man might suddenly feel stupid and inept. Let's have a little compassion here. If women find themselves unable to live up to the expectations of their own erotic imaginations, so do men, and they can't conceal their insecurities nearly as easily. To make this special party really happen, the "lucky" guy has to be at his best, emotionally as well as physically, since there's no spare dick to fill in for him should things get dicey. Strap-on dildos have their uses, but there is no substitute for the real thing. If you're that guy, you'll probably be playing all the porn scenes you've ever watched in your head and wondering how on earth you'll compete. It's easy to be overwhelmed by two sets of breasts and a couple of hungry pussies.

A friend of mine had been wanting a three-way forever. His girlfriend enlisted a very willing playmate, and they set out to show him a good time. To his chagrin and confusion, he never was able to perform sexually, though he did fuck his girlfriend like a champ after the guest had left. Why couldn't he step up to the opportunity of a lifetime? He didn't think he deserved it because he hadn't "made" it happen. Some men can receive sexual favors, and some men need to feel they are the initiators. Keep this in mind when determining how your encounter will begin. Some questions may be swirling around in his head. Who gets the attention? What happens if someone gets jealous? Will I be able to please both women, or will I be a total flop as a stud? What if they want each other more than they want me? We women have our worries, too, but there's little doubt which gender feels the most pressure in a threesome of this type.

Slaying the Dragons One at a Time

Who, exactly, does get the attention, anyhow? It's best to decide before you start. A basic strategy can help guide all of you past that awkward beginning. When my husband and I play with a woman, she's usually the focus of attention, since we're very experienced with threesomes and that's our preference. Sharing another woman is a special form of intimacy for us that we can get no other way. And attending to the guest first takes the pressure off him to come out of the starting gate with a porno-worthy erection. If the primary partner in an established couple is shy or the guest has more experience with women, then the female half of the couple would be the natural person with whom to begin. If the women are patient, especially if they're already friends, then the guy can be their initial point of connection. As things progress to more passionate interaction, who-gets-what-next will sort itself out more naturally. If both women are relatively inexperienced with bisexuality but game to experiment, I suggest they begin with necking and petting. Soon, arousal will take over, and hesitation will diminish.

Both men and women may have moments of jealousy, but that doesn't have to be a deal breaker, though it certainly can be. It may take several attempts at a threesome to resolve jealousy issues. I had my first threesome in my early twenties with my boyfriend of a couple of years and the first woman with whom I was ever sexual. I had dreamed of such an occasion for years and engineered it myself. Imagine my surprise when, very early on, I was overcome with a wave of jealousy and resentment that shocked me and upset them, bringing an abrupt end to the evening. While he and I never repeated that experiment and I didn't attempt it again for several more years, it was my

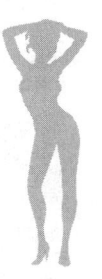

first object lesson in open sexuality. Jealousy arises out of our insecurities and indicates that some deeper need is going unmet. It's rarely about the other person, though we often project it onto him or her as a way to sidestep the real issue. Never ignore or deny jealous feelings. Take responsibility for your own reactions; your partner and/or guest can't read your mind. If you think someone is deliberately trying to inspire jealousy, call it a night and prepare for some tough conversation the morning after. As in any heavily charged discussion, forget shaming and blaming and stick to talking candidly about your own emotions. Very few useful sentences begin with the word *you*. It may be difficult, but loving communication goes a long way toward easing painful conflicts. If the verdict is "no more three-ways," so be it.

Are you "man enough" to satisfy two women? Thankfully, that's not entirely your responsibility. With all the superstud performances we see in porn, it's not surprising that a civilian dude may feel anus-clenching fear that he will somehow fall short of some arbitrary standard of excellence. The nervousness that naturally accompanies the realization of a long-held dream adds to the pressure. Never forget that movies are fantasy, with all the messy, awkward bits edited out for your sanitized viewing pleasure. While a hard cock is certainly part of the appeal, when it comes down to real people having real sex, the feelings generated among the three of you are much more important to the girls than a bit of anatomy over which you have no conscious control.

As you relax into the event and get over your shock that it's finally happening, your cock will generally rise to the occasion, if not to the proportions of a Titan rocket, though the overall success of the project doesn't depend on penile reliability. It may never get all the way hard on your first mission. Your erection comes and goes, often with no warning and for no apparent reason. You may be fine with your wife, but the condom makes it impossible to fuck the guest. If you get into that downward spiral of uneven performance leading to ever-greater anxiety, it may be difficult to make even a blow job work with the guest. After so much anticipation, you may be unable to keep yourself from coming sooner than you want. Your orgasm may prove elusive under such unfamiliar and challenging circumstances. Then again, you might amaze everyone and fuck both your partners like a stallion before shooting the biggest load of your life across four breasts or butt cheeks. At the end of the day (or evening), if you're having a good time, your playmates probably will as well. The threesome need not be a phallo-centric Olympiad to satisfy all the participants.

Then, of course, there is the fear of discovering that your mate is actually a lesbian. For some men, just being in the room while two women make love would be a dream come true, but for others it raises doubts that are probably unfounded. If one or both women have harbored same-sex fantasies for a long time, you can hardly blame them for being drawn in by the fascination of a first bisexual coupling. You've had more pussy than they have, so be magnanimous. If you can hang with it while they get to know each other, subsequent efforts will be more focused on you, as they move through the Rapture of the New into the realm of Sharing Our Boy Toy. Really.

While pussy is endlessly fascinating, as we all know, sooner or later your very maleness will be what's called for. Having an actual dick on hand is a powerful magnet for spare pussy. I've had more women since getting married than at any time in my life. As adaptable as women are and as skilled as I am, sometimes a girl still needs to get boned, and only a dude will do. If a playmate is not basically lesbian (and if she were, she probably wouldn't be at this particular party in the first

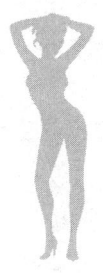

place), she'll need cock sooner or later, and won't you be happy that you waited your turn politely?

We Have Our Worries, Too

Even it it's something she's always wanted, a threesome raises as many anxieties for a woman as for a man, many of them overlapping. What if he finds her more attractive or sexier than he does me? How do I look naked by comparison? What if I'm no good at this? If I like touching her, will I end up spending the rest of my life in plaid shirts and Birkenstocks? If the other woman is a friend, will she still respect me in the morning?

Women have insecurities that are different from those of men when it comes to experimenting with bisexuality. We're taught to notice, criticize, and judge our appearance against that of our "rivals" for masculine attention. We're socialized to be both sisters under the skin as well as fierce competitors for the scarce resource of a "good man." Three-way sex breaches the territory of the primary partner, however enthusiastically she welcomed the idea, and there's bound to be some turbulence upon entry. The good news is many of these concerns resolve themselves. What I like best about the arithmetic of the BGG, as we call it in porn, is that it combines the warmth and intimacy of the strong, sisters-by-choice affection that is the hallmark of feminine culture with the satisfactions of enjoying a happy, grateful man. For the right two women such an arrangement, far from being a rank capitulation to "male privilege," feels surprisingly easy and natural, not to mention labor-saving. Which better girlfriend to dish to than she who also knows in the biblical sense the man you're talking about? Who better to send him to when you're not in the mood? Believe it or not, there are plenty of women and couples out there living this way right now. A threesome may be just an occasional treat, but it might also have the potential for a long-term alliance of mutual benefit.

If your main relationship is in good working order, as it should be before embarking on extracurricular activities, you already know how your partner feels about you and are secure in his affection. Believe me, no isolated or occasional time with another woman, no matter how earthshaking it may appear, holds out the dependable rewards of a healthy, committed relationship. As temporarily enthusiastic as my husband may get about a new playmate, I know through the experiences of a multiyear relationship where his true love and loyalty lie. He may like her a lot. He may want to fuck her a lot, but he doesn't want a serious relationship with anyone but me. We're the married couple, and our playmates are just passing through.

It can be disconcerting for your mate to exhibit the kind of supercharged attraction toward the extra player that he hasn't shown you since you were dating, but know that it's based on novelty and can't be sustained. Getting some "strange" will always carry an extra frisson of the mysterious and forbidden, but familiarity inevitably discharges much of the electricity. And don't forget that some of his very exuberance may stem from his satisfaction with you. Secure in your love and acceptance, he can allow himself to be fully present and exposed, as opposed to holding back and feeling uncertain. Take it as a compliment, if you can.

Mirror, Mirror, in my hand, who's the fairest in the land? This is the can of worms on the shelf labeled "jumbo extra crawly." Feminine insecurity regarding appearance is the bane of women everywhere, of every age, size, and shape. It incites countless, pointless arguments between

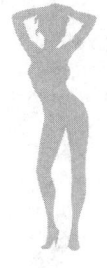

partners. Those little cultural voices reminding you that you're not a supermodel can't be totally silenced, but they needn't ruin your good time. In a hot triad situation, no one notices your supposed "figure flaw(s)." While you're lamenting the effects of gravity on your breasts, she's worrying about the spider veins in her thighs. Dress to feel comfortable and sexy, and then ditch the odious comparisons. Don't put yourself down, either silently or out loud. Learn to accept the compliments of your playmates graciously, no matter what counterarguments chatter in your mind. Believe me, they've got more important things to think about than whether or not you're carrying an extra ounce of cellulite.

One of the toughest challenges for women is initiating sexual contact, especially with each other. We're so used to our male lovers making the first move (that part of traditional male-female role assignment doesn't seem to have changed much) that we're often overcome by shyness when confronted with our first pair of breasts. You'll become a skilled lover of women with practice, just as you have with men. Touch another woman as you like to be touched. Kiss her as you like to be kissed. My first time kissing a woman was a revelation. No beard! So soft! So smooth! No wonder men like us so much; we're pretty adorable. The same approach applies to touching her pussy. Start with what works for you, or refer to the chapter on foreplay for women in this book for some tips. As a general rule, handle her more firmly than you're initially inclined. Once again, the touch that conveys confidence is the most effective.

Some of your female lovers will become friends and some won't. Some will remain friends after you're no longer lovers too. I've had plenty of threesomes none of us cared to repeat. They weren't unpleasant, but the personal chemistry didn't ignite. Other lovers have become so close that I ask them to visit my husband when I'm away on business, or I take them on weekend outings for just the two of us. If you like her without the sexual component, feel secure that she has her own life and that her involvement with you is all about good times rather than emotional dependency, the basic foundations of a sound friendship are there. If a potential partner seems at all unbalanced or too eager or has a chronically chaotic life, keep your distance. Learning to tell the difference between someone open to adventure and a potential future stalker takes practice. We're looking for girlfriends, not succubi. Some women like to foment discord within a relationship to make themselves feel powerful. Establish your intentions clearly from the start: play, good company, friendship, and fun, but no romance and no drama, thank you very much. Dragons now slain, we push on.

Creating Your Own Scenario

What kind of insurance can you devise to make your playdate successful? No measure of preparation absolutely guarantees success, but creative party planning can only help. My husband and I make lists of things we know our playmates like or can't get anywhere else, then add a surprise or two for that little thrill of unpredictability. We think in terms of mood and tone. Will the atmosphere be sensual, playful, or passionate? Will we segue from a candlelit dinner to a slow buildup, or strip down at the door for an afternoon of unabashed carnality? Is this to be a first-time thing, a one-time thing, or an ongoing thing? Taking all these factors into account, we lay out our blueprints accordingly.

If you're the host couple, set things up for your hot date ahead of time so that things flow smoothly once she's there. Any drinks or

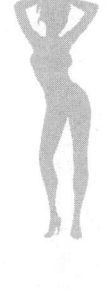

snacks should be set out, the CD player loaded with your preferred tunes, the phone turned off (after you've heard from her, of course!). In the bedroom all supplies should be laid out: condoms, gloves, lube, toys, and candles. It's also a good idea to take an extra flat sheet (dark is best, the better to hide lube stains) and place it over the bedspread. That way you won't have to change the sheets before going to sleep.

Having a plan to start with helps counteract any awkwardness when things are still new. Perhaps you'll dance while you have your glasses of wine and make like you're in high school as you pet and flirt. It's okay to be silly or nervous, so laugh all you need to. While you're still dressed you can kiss and hug and grind your hips to the beat, taking turns admiring one another. Three-way kisses fit in well here. Let the mood build naturally so you don't leave behind the one who's a little slower to get going. There are plenty of sexy, adult-themed board and dice games that can get the ball rolling. Strip poker is also a good bet. If you don't know how to play poker, strip go-fish is fine too. The key is to get comfortable with each other before proceeding. Two players kissing while the other one watches is very hot, especially if which two keeps changing.

If he is to be the center of attention, a two-woman sexy dance/kiss/strip is a surefire winner. With any luck, he'll get hard enough to wave his cock at both of you, which is a wonderful inspiration. Or one of you can sit in his lap and pet while the other one entertains you both. When she's peeled down to her scanties, she can trade places with you and enjoy the show you put on for them. By the time you get to your lingerie, he should be over any shyness and have plenty of ideas about what comes next. If he's bold, he can do a dance for the two of you, and before you know it you'll all be naked and ready for what's next.

If you and your partner have been thinking about this a long time and are very ready, making your guest the focus at first is a lovely experience for the woman as well as a way to keep you both closely connected to each other. One couple I knew was very good at tandem massage. No woman was immune to the combined ministrations of the two of them, and it proved a perfect way to get her out of her clothes! After a while, the action may become more two-way, or it can remain all about her the entire time. Some women are very comfortable receiving sensual pleasure, and others feel more secure in the giving mode. If you have one woman of each type at a threesome, you're good to go! If both women like to be active, he's a lucky man, indeed. If both like to be receptive, that's another kind of luck for him but also more work. Stay within your comfort zone so you don't freak out, but push yourself enough to keep it exciting. Finding that edge is where the heat is.

Perhaps you've invited a woman to play with you precisely because she's more experienced with women, and you and your partner want to take advantage of that fact. It's nice to let her take the lead. If she's any good, she'll be able to communicate what will happen next: "Let her rest her head in your lap while I take care of things down here," or "Let's both go down on him at the same time." Having one experienced person present can make all the difference between a party you want to repeat and one that you want to forget.

Doing the Math

When it gets down to it, what can you do with two pussies and one cock, six hands and three mouths? Plenty! While one person is eating, the other can be kissing. Being smothered in boobs while receiving oral sex is fantastic. Equally sexy is having someone sit on your face while another goes down on you. Talk about too much of a good thing! I like to put my mouth on one side of his hard cock, with

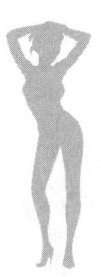

hers on the other side and French-kiss with him between us. It feels fantastic to everyone. Or, we can simply press our mouths along his shaft as he pumps between us, his hands on the backs of our heads. We can "fight" over his cock, taking a one-suck-for-you/one-suck-for-me approach. I also like to share cock-and-ball sucking duties: One will suck him while the other gives his scrotum a tongue bath. When doing tandem work, synchronize your efforts so that the stimulation is smooth rather than disjointed. If he's very advanced, she can lick behind his balls, too, or introduce a gloved finger to his butt (after prior consent, of course). The tried-and-true daisy chain is not to be discounted. He can eat her while she eats the other her, or he can get head and give it at the same time. If the players are limber enough, they might be able to complete the circle. It's unlikely that anyone can come like this as the distraction is too great, but it sure is fun!

When the fucking starts, the usefulness of the extra woman really stands out. One of my very favorite things to do is provide oral sex while two people are fucking. When they're spooning, I have access to everything, from both of their mouths to her clit, his butt, and back again, and I take full advantage of the smørgasbord, paying special attention to where his cock meets her pussy. Licking that margin sends them into orbit, I've found.

If they're in doggy, I can lie on my back and get head from her, or I can be behind him playing with his balls or butt or playing with her clit or holding a buzzing toy on it. If you do use your hands here, try pinching the shaft of her clit and letting the movement of the fucking do the rest, as opposed to trying to rub it too vigorously. Or simply press her clit onto her pubic bone and let the rocking of their bodies take care of the action. If he's wearing a condom, I like to squeeze the base bulb of his cock and provide as much skin-to-skin stimulation as possible. Also fun is to get in a 69 position, though you'll need a flat pillow to raise your head to crotch height to provide oral stimulation to them while they fuck. If 69ing won't work, get on your back with your feet going the same direction as theirs and get busy that way. Concentrate on using your mouth to provide his shaft with moist pressure. If you go for her clit, just latch on and suck; their body movements will do the rest, as your hands find something fun to do, whether it's playing with her breasts (nothing is more fun than bouncing boobs during doggy-style sex) or his balls and butt. The view's not bad, either—rather like being in a live porn tape.

If he's on his back, you can each straddle an end of him. It's easy to kiss each other this way and to play with boobs. If the women aren't bisexual, they don't have to touch each other. He'll be in heaven, certainly. One thing I love to do when she's in cowgirl is to get between their legs and provide manual assistance. I can slip a gloved finger into one or both of their butts, provide clitoral pressure with a spare hand, play with his balls and scrotum and massage her pussy while he's in her as well as smack her butt cheeks.

Missionary is good, too, as it turns out. If he's fucking her, I can sit on her face and he and I can kiss. Or, if I bend over from there, he can rest his head on my back for a very cozy moment while I hold her legs up or pull her knees back. I also like to lie beside them and take it all in while I play with her boobs, kiss them both, hold her hand, provide clitoral assistance, or masturbate myself. My all-time favorite thing to do is to get between their legs and again put my hands to good use. Gloved fingers in butts, of course, and ball play, but there's a lot more to do. It feels fantastic (unless it's distracting, in which case they need to tell you) when you rub her *fourchette* and the sides of her introitus as he fucks her. It spreads the sensation around deliciously. Methodically run your fingers back and forth from the four-o'clock position to

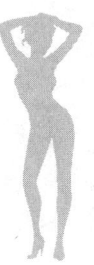

the eight-o'clock position over and over again or use two hands, one on either side of his cock, to knead her flesh. From there, it's easy and natural for a finger to slip into her pussy along the bottom of his cock. Face the finger up, and it's a wonderful added pressure on him. Face it down, and it's a fantastic PC muscle massage/stretch for her. If there's room, slip two fingers in, one on either side of his shaft. Facing up, with your palm cupping his balls, you'll feel the head of his cock slide between your fingers and you can use your thumb to massage the bulb of his penis. On the out-stroke, bend your fingers, and you'll massage her G-spot. If you face your fingers down, you'll slide into her posterior fornix for extra oomph. Be sure to coordinate your moves with their fucking, so your efforts are an enhancement instead of an annoyance. End up with as many fingers in as feels good to her.

In the beginning, it's useful to agree ahead of time where and with whom he'll come. Until you feel very confident, you may want him to finish off with you, just to keep the bond tight. Or you may have always wanted to see him shoot on a woman's breasts, or to witness another woman's oral technique, or to be kissing him while he fulfills his fantasy of coming with another woman. If he's having trouble with condoms, his orgasm likely will be via fellatio or masturbation, but that's pretty hot, too.

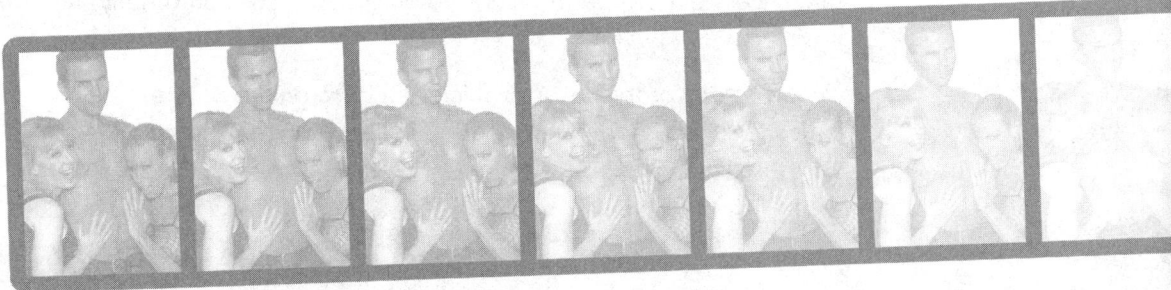

TRIANGULAR TOPPERS

1 • *Let the girls take the lead.* Whether close friends or new acquaintances, it's going to be pretty much their show, and they should decide when the curtain goes up.

2 • *Start slow.* Making out, slow stripping, playful flirting, and casually hanging out in the nude give you all a chance to get comfortable before taking the plunge.

3 • *Before anyone makes a move, be sure the limits are absolutely clear* regarding who has permission to do what to whom. It may take a couple of dates prior to anyone doing anything just to set these boundaries.

4 • *If the women are to interact sexually, especially if neither is otherwise actively bisexual, take extra care to be certain both are equally willing.* Two against one is bad math for all.

5 • *Allow plenty of time to get physically acquainted.* With three bodies to explore, two of them female, there's no such thing as too much foreplay.

6 • *Once things get serious, be inclusive without insisting.* Always acknowledge the presence of the third party, even if only two are directly engaged at a given moment. Sitting back and watching, or being watched, is part of the payoff.

7 • *Expect some awkward moments.* The geography is more complex than usual, and you won't initially interact with the ball-bearing smoothness of porn performers who do group scenes on a daily basis.

8 • *Deal with any problems or conflicts that arise on the spot,* even if it means cutting short your hot date. Better disappointment now than resentment later.

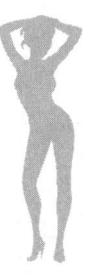

THREE-WAY SPLITS

1 • *No spur-of-the-moment experiments.* Tempting as it might be to invite a partner's best friend to "stay over" after a couple of drinks, you'll be happier in the long run if you talk it over sober and make a specific playdate.

2 • *It's not all about dick.* While in the common male fantasy of two-girl threesomes, the gals act like a pair of horny houris from *I Dream of Jeannie,* they're there as much for themselves and each other as they are for him.

3 • *No nagging, whining, bribing, guilt tripping, or other manipulative tactics to persuade a reluctant third.* You'll be deservedly embarrassed if she rejects you and even worse off if she pretends not to just so you'll shut up about it.

4 • *Never consent to a threesome just because a primary partner wants it.* You may be acting out of generosity or desperation, but either way you'll all regret it later.

5 • *Forget about "satisfying" everybody's needs in every possible way.* Attentions will naturally be divided, and the pleasures may not be evenly distributed on any given occasion. It may take more than one attempt to strike the correct balance.

6 • *Do not, on the other hand, neglect your S.O. in your fascination with your newfound fuck buddy.* It's rude and will discourage closer encounters of the third kind.

7 • *No competition among the players.* This is a team sport; showing off for the benefit of a fresh audience rarely makes a good impression on anybody.

8 • *No boasting after the fact.* Spare your watercooler mates your version of *Penthouse* "Forum." As in Vegas, what goes on in your bedroom stays there. Remember that axiom about the six degrees of separation.

Chapter 14

THREE-WAY SEX:
TWO GUYS AND A GIRL—
AS MUCH FUN AS IT SOUNDS

Men would be surprised to know how many women fantasize about having sex with two of them at the same time. While depictions of three-way sex involving two women and one man are common in our media culture, the inverse equation is far less frequently seen, outside the world of porn, at least. But some of the same elements that make the concept of a simultaneous coupling with two women so appealing to men apply equally when the equation is reversed. The thrill of the unfamiliar, the prospect of receiving the simultaneous attentions of two partners at once, and the sheer anatomical abundance of the situation stimulate the feminine imagination just as effectively. Likewise, in contemplating the actualization of such a scenario, many of the same fears and insecurities arise. Will I be able to

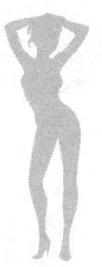

satisfy both? How can I communicate my own wants and needs when I'm outnumbered? What impact will the encounter have on my existing relationships? Am I ready to know whatever I may discover about myself in the process?

Unlike my disastrous initial three-way with another woman, my first taste of sex with two men went down easy, an experience I've since discovered isn't all that uncommon. My then-boyfriend and I had a happily experimental sexual relationship in which we shared many of our previously secret desires. We'd already lived out the one involving a second woman, and with great results. When his best friend from high school came through town, conditions seemed ideal. Once the guys had talked it through and were sure it wouldn't mess up their friendship, the date was on, and I was ready. We booked a motel room and brought what meager supplies we had: lube, condoms, and some candles. We socialized a bit as we sipped some drinks, but the situation was, admittedly, a bit awkward at the beginning. Who was supposed to make the first move? My partner suggested that I kiss his friend. While I was enjoying that, my boyfriend started to caress me, I put my hands on his friend, and all went smoothly from there. The first move may be the hardest, but nature will take over once the touching begins.

Having four hands and two mouths on me at once was intoxicating, as was having my hands around two eager cocks. My most vivid memory, though, is of my own happy surprise at how comfortable we all were with one another. It felt completely natural for my boyfriend to fuck me from behind while I enjoyed a hard cock in my face. I really liked being eaten out by one while I sucked the other. The sensations of new lips on my pussy and a familiar dick in my hand were intoxicating. It was even more fun to play with both penises at the same time, going back and forth, just like in the porn movies I'd already started watching and would someday make. The whole evening was a particularly daring romance novel come to life. Playing with so much confident, sexually relaxed masculinity was profoundly liberating. With no competition between them, my two dates were free to focus their erotic energy on me. For once, my sexual appetite didn't seem excessive. We had an exhausting but entirely enjoyable evening together. We never did it again, but I remember the experience fondly to this day, and it's been more than twenty years! I don't know what happened to my playmates thereafter, as we drifted apart, but I'm still grateful to them for the opportunity they provided.

You Truly Can Have It All

The conventional unconventional wisdom holds that a first three-way experience will likely be among two women and a man. Our culture certainly encourages us to regard such a configuration as closer to "normal," since this less-challenging, male-centered sexual fantasy is more commonly seen in both adult entertainment and mainstream media. However, as women have become more assertive in sharing their erotic desires and men have opened their imaginations to pursuing different varieties of sexual fulfillment, the concept of two men enjoying a single woman has grown in acceptance. As we've noted, group-sex exploration usually begins with an inquisitive couple adding one more player. Contrary to the social construction of three-way sex, not all sexually adventurous women are bisexual, and many men find the idea of watching a woman have sex with another man every bit as appealing as watching the same activities between two women. Indeed, the healthy sales of boy-girl porn to a primarily male audience would sug-

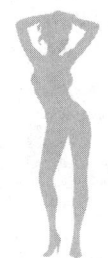

gest that this is the kind of sex most men prefer to see. For many men and women, the two-man/one-woman play party is as natural a fit as the two-woman version is for other couples. But getting from fantasy to reality may require a bit more patience and ingenuity, and a bit more stage managing, than would simply luring your best gal pal into a birthday romp with your S.O. after a festive dinner.

It takes a brave woman to tell her partner she wants sex with another man, just as it takes a very secure man to accept his beloved's desire for another dick, even if only every now and then. Conflict and distress over fantasies and desires are very common among women, as issues of "purity," "chastity," and "virtue" come back unexpectedly to haunt them, even after they've convinced themselves of their own liberated modernity.

In addition to this emotional baggage, there are practical concerns that can never be too far from any woman's mind. A sexually unconventional woman often fears she'll never find a mate, leaving many to waste years in relationships that deny key elements of their intimate identities. While most women are happy to love just one man and smart enough to focus their romantic attentions on a worthy mate, not all women are cut out to be physically monogamous, however deeply they love their husbands. Many keep quiet for years about their need for additional cock, fearing they'll be judged greedy, perverted, slutty, shallow, or, worst of all, compulsively unfaithful. Even today, women often lack the sense of entitlement when it comes to sexual pleasure that society has historically granted to men. Only by allowing themselves the same curiosities and possibilities as men do can women be truly equal partners in the bedroom, and that's the kind of partner a wise man desires.

The B Word

There is a cultural tendency to pathologize the desire for sex among two men and one woman. Is such a wish really evidence of (heaven forefend!) covert male bisexuality? Does it suggest weaknesses and inadequacies in existing relationships? Isn't it all just a show to satisfy the voyeurism of the guys?

Many men tell me of their appreciation for their female partners' robust sexual appetites and find the idea of watching their mates at play with other men to be very hot but are hesitant to act on the prospect because it seems "gay." Trust me, the mere presence of another penis in the room, or in your wife, doesn't automatically invalidate a lifetime of heterosexuality. Any man who wants this kind of sex just has to get over himself in this area, one way or another.

For some men, a three-way encounter involving a second male participant carries no gender-identity implications whatsoever. Under these ground rules, both men are there because of the woman. Their energies are focused on her, and the sex is with her. The opportunity for straight men to bond closely, even emotionally, through the body of the woman is a sort of social bonus, like playing a team sport. I've been that woman many times and can testify to the satisfaction found at the nexus where true affection between confident, heterosexual men finds expression. Experiencing masculine desire absent masculine competition is very exciting in itself, and an aroused female has no trouble focusing the arousal of two straight men. With any luck, they'll be much too busy to worry about being naked in front of each other. Watching one's sweetheart suck cock while fucking her doggy-style definitely beats out video porn any day.

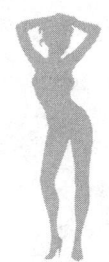

To say that there is never erotic energy between two men in such a situation, however, is to lie, since plenty of men are "bi-curious" themselves. Just as the presence of a man makes it easier for a woman to experiment with another woman, so, too, does the presence of a woman make it easier for a man to explore his homoerotic fantasies without surrendering his het status.

As millions of women will attest, cock sucking is fun, so why should we have a monopoly on it? Some women pursue bisexual men as ardently as some men I know court bisexual women. I've met more than a few couples that love to suck dick together, in between the men taking turns fucking her. The bond between couples that have forged such compatible matches has the tensile strength of Swedish steel. Contrary to what we're so often told, such unconventional matches have always existed and are no more or less normal than any other kind.

At the end of the day (or in the middle of the afternoon, if that's more convenient), unanimous consensus, created by open and honest communication, is the only acceptable standard. What brought you together is ultimately less important than what you do once you're there. You'll create your own version of normal, which may be utterly heterosexual or casually inter-gendered, and that's the one that counts.

To Build a Great Trio, Start with a Strong Duet

Getting past "What if . . . ?" to "Wow, I'm actually doing this!" requires determination, creativity, and, most important, fearless candor with yourself and others, before and after the fact. It's going to take some doing before everybody ends up getting done, and that process begins at home. No matter who you are or what previous experience you bring to the mix, certain basic emotional dynamics will predictably be in play.

It's natural for a man whose partner expresses a wish for sex with another guy to have some concerns, even if the fantasy appeals. His doubts are just as valid as her desires and deserve just as much respect from both before they move on to the next step. In the context of a primary relationship, the male partner needs to know he'll still be number one, no matter how much fun his spouse has with their playmate. And it's natural for a woman to entertain doubts about her own attractiveness and her partner's long-term reliability if he's the one who initiates the discussion. You both need to set emotional boundaries around your involvement with an outsider and to observe them scrupulously. Your trust in each other must be solid, or the introduction of a third party may open stress fractures between you that will be difficult, if not impossible, to mend.

Most people don't ever get to this line, much less cross it, leaving those who do to chart their own courses. The place to start is where you're standing. If a man doesn't find the idea of sharing his girl genuinely exciting and plays along only to please her, or to avoid losing her, the results will be disappointing at best. At worst, you'll all have a bad time, and his deepest fears will be realized anyway. Better he should decline to participate and step up to the consequences of his refusal. Similarly, rather than allow herself to be used as boy bait by a bisexual spouse in denial, a woman would be better off to make a three-way date with Rover and a divorce lawyer. The only legitimate reason to experiment with multipartner sex of any kind is a sincere, personal desire to do so. All other motives are tainted by manipulation, which is the most common and most damaging sin against responsible non-monogamy.

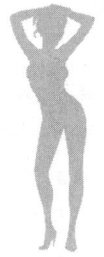

Even if an existing couple has a common interest in pursuing such an experiment, the timetable can't be rushed. While either partner can certainly encourage his or her mate to consider the possibilities, nagging, whining, heavy-handed hinting, leaving your favorite all three-ways all the time, four-hour compilation video in the sock drawer and other pressure tactics won't lead to anything good.

The confidence needed to attempt feats of sexual daring only grows in an atmosphere of acceptance, including acceptance of the right to say "no" or "maybe later" without fear of rejection. Bottom line: Unless the woman finds the prospect of a dick in each hand exciting and the man can masturbate to the idea of his wife being fucked by two men at once, better to give the whole package a pass.

Above all, before an established couple invites others to the party, they need to feel confident of one another's loyalty and affection. However the attempt turns out, they must be certain they'll be happy going home together. It's also reassuring to the potential third partner to know that, emotionally, the woman isn't dissatisfied with her primary relationship and looking for romance. It's more flattering and less threatening for him to see himself as a treat for a happy, self-confident couple than it would be for him to feel as if he's a life preserver for a relationship circling the drain. If the man in question has difficulty grasping this concept, he's not qualified for the job.

Man Wanted

If a hard man is good to find, finding two of them who can work and play well together with one woman is a real challenge. He doesn't need to be Mr. Right (presumably, you've already found that guy), but he does have to be Mr. Right-for-the-Occasion, and he may prove elusive at first. Just remember, you cannot go forward until you're both confident you've chosen the correct third leg for your triangle.

Some of the same social dynamics that determine the success or failure of an encounter among two women and one man apply in this search, and some don't. A close friend of either gender, for instance, might be an obvious candidate for triad play, and similar considerations regarding respect for the existing friendship would certainly be important. The close friend may be a bit too close, especially if what's proposed would fundamentally redefine the friendship. If one guy's best pal is secretly in love with the woman in question, this is a very unwise way to find out about it. Similarly, an old boyfriend of the female participant might be a perfect choice for this situation, or he might stir up old feelings better left dormant.

Both men and women can be competitive and insecure about sex in ways they don't realize until put to the test of exploring sexuality outside the box. These issues need to be discussed in advance of any physical experimentation, lest valuable associations be put in jeopardy. And there may prove to be one particularly awkward difference in dealing with two men as opposed to two women. Cultural taboos make it excruciatingly difficult for men to talk about their feelings. A woman pursuing a satisfying threesome may need to act as a conversational facilitator first, opening up about her emotional responses and inviting the men to do likewise. Be prepared for the possibility of arriving at "no" instead of "yes."

Wouldn't it be safer to try it with a stranger? This depends on what kind of safety we're talking about. A stranger may not bring the complications of an existing relationship to the mix, but he might have other drawbacks. While he does add the appeal of the unknown, until or unless you and your partner are very experienced in three-way play,

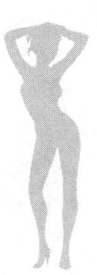

I would be very hesitant about taking home that seemingly nice guy the two of you met at a bar. He could be great, a big disappointment, or, at worst, even a danger. At the very least, make sure you ask lots of questions and get a hotel room instead of taking him to your home.

Organized swinging groups or functions may prove amenable to this kind of search, since by definition the people that attend are (1) interested in talking openly about sex, and (2) often into multipartner sex. Also, by the time a man gets to a swing party, he may have prior experience with the two-guy/one-gal setup. Swinging men are mainly heterosexual, but they've worked through a lot of their other issues about public sex and nudity. Given the frequency of the common two-woman/one-guy triad at swing events, there are often spare husbands available for the other three-way combo. There has been some relaxation of the swinging world's notorious homophobia in recent years, and swinging men are very welcoming of a woman's sexual stamina and desire, finding it one of the most rewarding things about the Lifestyle.

At swing parties, you may certainly be able to get the male half of a couple to spend some time with you in the group room, but you won't be alone together. However, if the extra guy's female partner is secure enough not to need to be in the room or is diverted by her own activities, you may find a private space for your fun. So, polyamory-friendly environments where people understand the rules of the game are often good venues for getting together with unfamiliar players. Established rules of conduct help strangers and novices navigate the tricky waters of sexual negotiation. Even if these situations don't offer exactly what you're looking for, they make for entertaining and informative field studies and might be good starting points.

The Internet has become a vibrant market for the pursuit of sexual variety, and there are many sites, chat rooms, and user groups devoted to every permutation of multipartner activity. But modern technology doesn't eliminate the need for the caution and common sense you would have exercised in response to a printed personals ad a decade ago. It's very easy for people to misrepresent themselves or simply fail to make themselves understood in the incorporeal ether of cyberspace. There are potential dangers lurking out there but, more commonly, potential disappointments and embarrassments. A bit of healthy skepticism toward claims made in electronic forums may avoid unwanted outcomes down the line.

However you make the acquaintance of your outside man, the protocols for what happens next remain essentially the same. All first meetings should be in public places. Full names, addresses, and occupations need to be shielded until at least rudimentary trust is established. Then, for the safety of all, they must be shared. Anonymity carries risks of its own. Full disclosure of your sexual histories and your long-term intentions (if any) is ethically required. Limits need to be negotiated in detail, especially with a socially unfamiliar third party. Take nothing for granted. Talk about everything. It won't help to pretend to be more experienced than you are. A worthwhile contender will be willing to put in the extra time and effort needed to ensure the good experience sought by all. If you're still uncertain after that second meeting, you probably need to move on. If you do decide to go forward with a mutually chosen outsider, do so with the awareness that getting to know someone in this way is an unpredictable process, possibly requiring you all to enforce your rules more vigorously than expected or even to get up and leave if the feeling isn't right. And in any sexual encounter with a stranger, rigorous safe-sex precautions must be religiously observed. Denial can be deadly when it comes to three-ways involving two men. STDs are more easily transmitted man-to-woman or man-to-

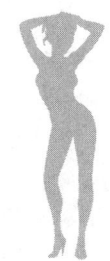

man, so keep those condoms handy and don't forget to use them. Fast and accurate STD testing is now available to the public in most large cities, and particularly for this type of play, a trip to the local clinic, unsexy as it sounds, may be the best prelude to a relaxed, worry-free party. While awaiting the test results (which will take several days), you can engage your ingenuity by playing the "What can we do that's sexy and safe?" game. Many warm long-term friendships have started this way.

One of the frustrations of giving sound, common-sense advice about unconventional sex is knowing that much of it will be ignored. As with more common two-woman threesomes, couples who can't, or won't, look their desires for multipartner sex in the eye will often resort to the "have a few drinks together and see what happens" approach. Changing the arithmetic doesn't change the odds. While this strategy very occasionally results in a not-so-bad night, the odds are greatly improved by better planning. At the very least, before proceeding, everyone needs to know what he or she does and doesn't want. You can always change the rules later if you become more comfortable together and feel more daring. At the outset, be as specific as you need to, and don't mince words. You'll be pleasantly surprised at all your mutual relief when the particulars are made clear and the guesswork is over. If a couple can't articulate their part of the deal, they're not ready for this kind of party. Once the boundaries are drawn, there will be plenty of room for spontaneity in private.

Some Assembly Required

Nature gives a woman everything she needs to handle two men at once, and she'll need everything she's got. The woman can expect to work a little harder for both men to receive their fair share of her attention, so the more confidently she can express feminine desire as well as receptivity, the more she'll get what she wants from both men. She'll be kept pretty busy and shouldn't hesitate to let both her partners experience her appreciation. With a bit of imagination and a willingness to please, one woman can be a great date for two men. Two-guy threesomes are the perfect setup for an energetic, creative woman with a healthy appetite for sex. She'll have the starring role in her own personal movie.

There are lots of little, practical things to keep in mind to make such a gathering work smoothly. Remember you're giving a party here, even if the guest list is short. Make sure you have plenty of time and plenty of privacy. If this means renting a hotel room, book the nicest one you can swing. Be sure to dress conservatively in public spaces, and it helps to behave conventionally. Wait until you're in private before turning playful. When you check in, ask for extra towels, washcloths, etc. Bring candles or scarves to create atmosphere. It might be nice to bring a CD player for music, but it's best if it's not too loud. Make sure whatever toys, baby wipes, favorite lubes, condoms, gloves, or other supplies you need are conveniently available. Don't forget the extension cord for the vibrator! As for intoxicants, I've found the fewer the better. There is no pleasure in having sex while drunk or with someone who's drunk, and there's certainly no sport in it! Besides, drunk men can't fuck, and drunk women can't take care of anybody. This kind of sex requires your full attention. If a glass of wine helps you all relax, no problem, but you'll want to be in possession of your senses to fully appreciate the experience, so stop at two. Keep the noise level down; nothing breaks the mood more quickly than a visit from security telling you that "we've had some complaints about the noise from your room."

There's bound to be awkwardness the first time, so cut everybody some slack. Your results may depart from the freewheeling tumbles you see in videos. Any of you might not know that he or she is jealous

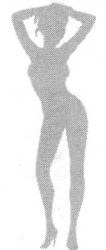

or insecure until confronted with those feelings in the middle of the action. If such conflicts arise, the person having them needs to say: "Let's slow down for a minute." Often, just a moment of quiet as the individual calms down is all that's needed. As a practical tip, when returning to sex play after such a break, go back to the last thing you were doing that was comfortable for everyone and take it from there. It's never advisable to ignore emotional signals during sex.

Start slow, with lots of teasing and foreplay. The lucky girl can do a sexy dance for the two guys, letting loose her inner stripper. This puts the focus on her and lets her direct the action. She can fondle both crotches at once or fondle one while she uses her mouth on the other.

If the guys are straight, it's really all about the woman, so she can let herself off the leash to follow her pleasure and desire. The men get to watch a porn movie and be in it at the same time. For the woman, there's nothing quite like being fucked while she has another dick to suck. So much man! Really, it's delicious. Don't rush. Do the easiest things first and see what develops. Unlike pros, you're not making a movie, so don't be too goal oriented. Let things unfold naturally instead of pushing for acrobatics. In porn, it's our job to make everything look easy and natural, but for folks at home, everything needs to actually *be* easy and natural, or it's not worth the effort. Keep in mind that it isn't necessary for all three partners to be equally engaged at all times. Kicking back and watching can be exciting too. Don't assume that a dick in every hole at all times is the measure of a successful threesome.

With the preliminaries out of the way, what's on the menu? Here are some basic combinations to get you started: The woman can kneel between the men, playing with and sucking each cock in turn. They can jerk off in her face while she masturbates to the hot sight or fondles their balls. She can straddle them as they lie on the bed or sit on the edge, going back and forth between them. Using only my hands, I like to practice my ambidexterity by doing exactly the same thing to each penis in exactly the same manner to see how they respond. With one guy on his back, the woman can sit on him while she sucks the other. By facing the feet of the man she's fucking, she can keep enough distance between the men to avoid potentially uncomfortable man-to-man contact, and the guy on the bottom has a great view of her ass as well as the oral action.

Certainly, the easiest position is doggy-while-sucking-the-other-partner. It's also fun to suck one guy while the other eats pussy or uses a toy or hand to stimulate the female player. If there is to be anal play, be sure to use latex gloves for *any* contact, to avoid accidental cross-contamination. By replacing the gloves religiously, hands stay clean without the need to hop up and go wash.

If the men are game, they can try double-vaginal penetration: The "anchor" lies on his back, and the woman gets on top of him, facing forward. The second man kneels behind and slips his dick into her. For obvious reasons, this is not for everyone, but the ones who have tried it say it's incredibly hot and sexy. In this same basic position, if anal sex is desired, the man in back can put his dick into her butt instead of her pussy. Be very careful not to let lube drip from her butt, or she may get a nasty infection as a souvenir.

It might take more than one soiree to get it all going. Don't be discouraged if your first three-way date ends up with a double blow job, two hand jobs, or three-way masturbation. This isn't a competitive sport or a contest about penis size or hard-ons. Learning to be sexually relaxed around another man requires some practice. Erections may come and go. Orgasms and ejaculations may prove elusive. Just remember that this is about the journey, not the destination.

It may take time for all of you to get comfortable enough for actual

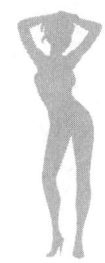

intercourse. Making the transition from fantasy to reality can be tricky, and we must give ourselves plenty of space to be human. Different people make their accommodations to alternative sexual expression at different rates. It may be months between the first attempt and the next, while the primary couple works out the dynamics. The more-comfortable partner needs to be patient and encouraging while the less-comfortable partner figures out what's what.

Becoming sexually intimate with another person is never a light or trivial matter, so give it the respect it deserves. Your threesome will be a product of what you all bring to it. And what you get out of it will depend on how honest and responsible you are in the way you treat one another.

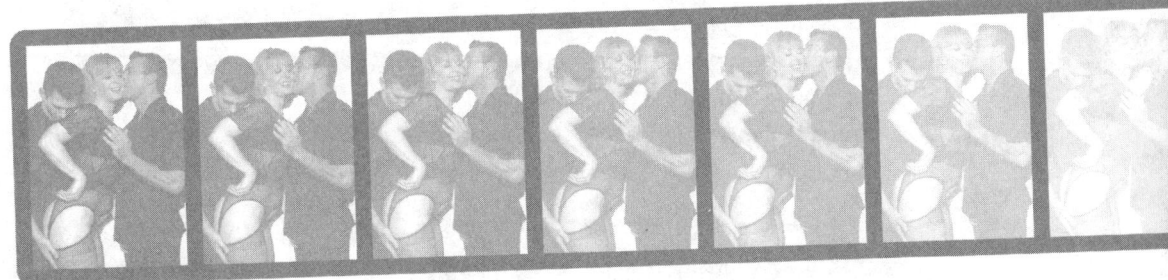

TWO-ON-ONE TEMPTATIONS

1 • *Do your homework.* Plenty of discussion beforehand with your mate helps clear up doubts, establish ground rules, and set standards for an experience you can all enjoy.

2 • *Be picky.* It's going to require a very special man to make himself at home with an established couple. Look beyond appearances to good manners, sexual sophistication, and a willingness to talk openly and in detail about what you all hope to get out of your experience together.

3 • *Try a social occasion first.* If you're all compatible over dinner, that's a good start. An unpressured evening together gives you all a chance to scope one another out and make an informed decision before you're all naked in a room someplace.

4 • *Make a plan and stick with it.* Once you're sure you're all on the same page and really ready to proceed, don't dissipate the charge with vague promises and unnecessary rescheduling. If anyone experiences real reservations, call off your date and have done with it; otherwise, make it happen.

5 • *Lay out your game plan in advance.* Settle on a date, an hour, a place, and any specific enhancements you all want to include. Clear the decks at home or wherever you're going to play, and lay in whatever refreshments, toys, music, costumes, etc., you think you might want. Remember that with three people, you'll need plenty of lube, gloves, condoms, and other basic supplies so nobody has to make a drugstore run in the middle.

6 • *When it's time, it's time.* Once you're together for your hot session, all questions should have been answered and doubts addressed, so don't be coy. Believe me, after you all get busy, you'll be grateful for every available moment.

7 • *Unlike the waltz, when it comes to two-guy three-ways, the woman always leads.* She can initiate the party with a bit of hot dancing, an impromptu strip, or just going straight for the zippers, but if she doesn't make the first move, the guys may be too shy.

8 • *Take your time.* Until you've played this way repeatedly, the anatomical permutations may seem a bit clumsy for all. Let the scene unfold at a natural, unhurried pace while you get comfortable with one another.

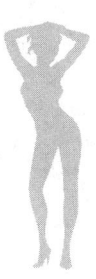

9 • *Honor thy deal.* Whatever limits you all put in place during the negotiation phase, observe them rigorously in your actual play. As your level of experience rises, you may feel more comfortable improvising, but at first, agreed rules, especially concerning safer sex, make everyone feel more secure.

10 • *Stay in touch.* While distracting talk may spoil the mood, matters of physical discomfort or emotional distress need immediate attention. Likewise, letting your partners know what's working for you is the best way to get more of it.

Troubles for Trios

1 • *Don't proceed without a truly unanimous vote.* It's all too easy for two people to subtly intimidate or manipulate a less-than-completely-willing third party. Make sure everybody's truly up for the game, or call it rained out.

2 • *Resist the temptation to rush into something with an unfamiliar playmate.* Beware the appealing stranger who might turn out to be quite different in private from the man you met in the bar. Impulsive decisions can lead to unpleasant outcomes.

3 • *Never ignore your own cautionary instincts.* If, for whatever reason, any one of you feels the time isn't right, better to call it off than to proceed reluctantly.

4 • *No hidden agendas.* This type of group situation is particularly prone to bad outcomes resulting from failure to disclose bisexual interests or the lack thereof. Do not wait until everybody's naked to disclose basic differences.

5 • *Avoid any tendency to make your threesome into a competitive event.* Certainly both men will be out to please the woman, but they shouldn't try to outdo each other at doing her.

6 • *Don't say yes when your body says no.* Two excited men can be a bit much for one woman. If any anatomical parts start feeling overworked, give them a rest. Your body will thank you for it the day after.

7 • *No pairing off without prior agreement.* Some men really do prefer to watch and masturbate while the other two lovebirds do the mating dance. More frequently, however, a significant imbalance in erotic attentions leads to jealousy, hurt feelings, and bad memories. You're all in this together, from start to finish.

8 • *Never get so carried away in the heat of the moment that you forget who's been where and in what order.* Socket switching is part of the appeal of double-dick situations, but proper sanitary technique is a must to avoid needless trips to the doctor's office. Just keep changing those condoms and gloves.

9 • *Don't reveal any deep, dark secrets you may discover about one another to outsiders.* It's a very small world, populated by some very small-minded people. It's unethical to expose a playmate to the possible social consequences of your need to brag.

10 • *No recriminations after the fact.* Everything was done by mutual consent. Doubts, insecurities, and suggestions for next time should be shared with the utmost tact, as raw and unfamiliar emotions may be brought to the surface by the power of new experiences.

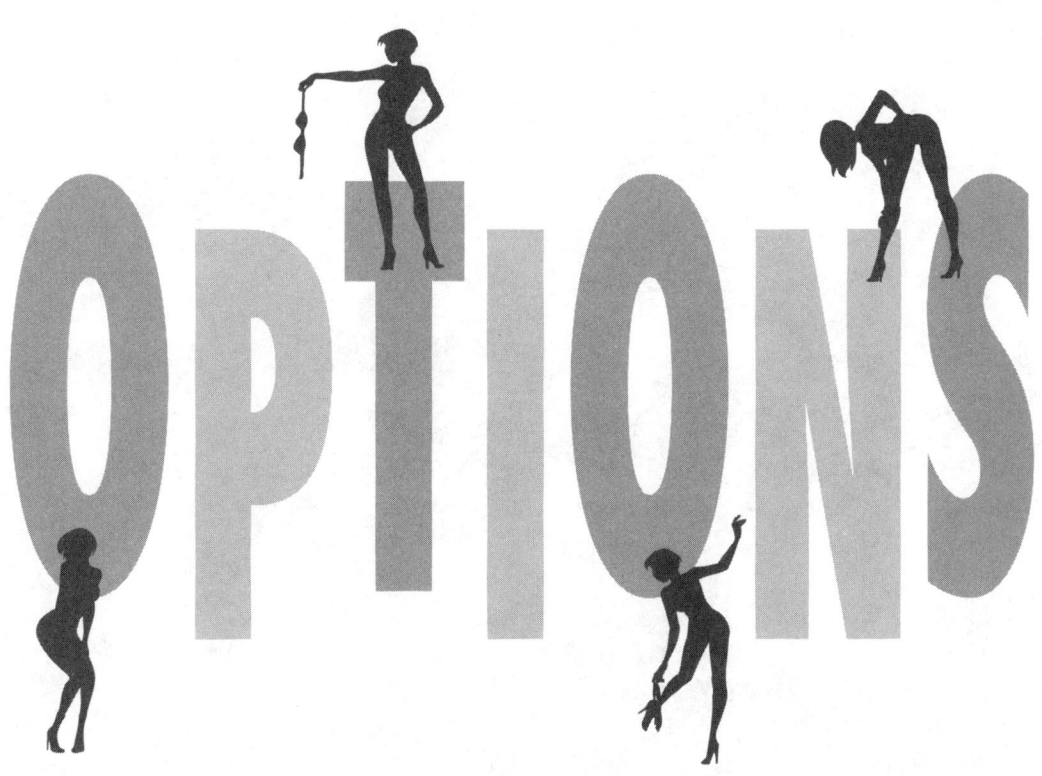

Chapter 15

SENSUAL DOMINATION: TAKING CONTROL

'm sure I'm not the only one to notice the emergence of props and costumes from the demimonde of what used to be called "S&M" and their entrance into the cultural mainstream. I see leather, whips, chains, collars, blindfolds, corsets, bondage gear, and other fetishistic totems in advertising, music videos, and even sit-coms so frequently, I find myself wondering if the whole world has gone kink overnight or if the clever folks who create media products haven't merely latched on to a touch of taboo to give their work a frisson of the forbidden. Beneath the visual cues lies a fascinating dream world of erotic power exchange that we may visit as often as we like for as long as we like, once we've found the map that gets us there. My moment of illumination came when I recognized that the dominant and submissive scenarios in which we engage are really extended forms of foreplay that directly connect our fantasy lives with the realities of our sexual experiences.

It's nearly impossible to discuss the enmeshed relationship between sex and power without touching the third rail. For most of human history, one gender has been conditioned to exercise power whenever and wherever possible, including sexually, while the other gender has been conditioned to accept this grudgingly and resist it only by indirection. In Western culture, this conventional wisdom has been stood on its head during the past century, with both genders being told that the personal is political and that any exercise of power in a sexual context is inherently an act of oppression.

There is something real behind the confusion we experience. However conventional a sexual encounter may appear, and even if the people involved don't know it, power is being exchanged at all times in a spoken or implicit contract of How It's Going to Be Between Us. What sets conscious power players apart from our nonkinky friends is that we openly acknowledge, accept, embrace, fetishize, and sexualize this fact, bringing it to the forefront of our discussions and negotiations with potential partners.

Again, we see how little politics helps us in the bedroom. No matter how loudly church, state, and the women's studies program at the local university may thunder at us about the evils inherent in our yearning to combine the volatile forces of sexual desire and the will to power, that yearning persists in both men and women. Because of what I do for a living, people talk to me about their inner sex lives as they might hesitate to talk to a psychiatrist or a priest, much less a spouse. From my admittedly anecdotal and unscientific observations, I can only conclude that the hunger for some form of sexual power exchange

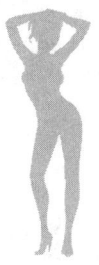

is as common among both men and women as the equally taboo and exciting urge for sex with a stranger. No matter how stridently we're told not to want these things, vast numbers of us still do.

Even if you never choose to act out your own fantasies of sexual domination, it behooves you to recognize, understand, and accept them. That which you deny in yourself doesn't just go away. It operates in secret, influencing your behavior and your life decisions in ways you can neither comprehend nor control. Coming to terms with your own conflicts about sex and power is the best protection from their unwanted emergence in inappropriate circumstances.

So let's just go ahead and peek from behind intertwined fingers at the possible origins of those spectral images of yourself in command of your sex partner that haunt you as he or she sleeps next to you at night. Are you a bad person for wanting, at least momentarily, someone you love to surrender to your wishes—demands even—and derive his or her erotic satisfaction from serving yours? If you are, you've certainly got lots of company. It's not for nothing that images of erotic domination, amazons in thigh-high boots, and leather-clad biker dudes are so prevalent in our popular culture. Absent highbrow pretensions of taste and class, popular culture reflects our collective id, which is where these archetypes that become stereotypes and finally media clichés reside.

I've listened to every argument insisting that the pull of erotic domination is socially constructed, just as I have to those equally persuasive views that they are innate and immutable. Neither absolutist interpretation squares neatly with my own instinct and experience, which tell me that, without aggression, there would be no sexual desire, no sex, no procreation, and, ultimately, no life. Every living thing must compete with every other to sustain itself and to reproduce its kind. Without that pure, dark drop of intraspecies aggression, the competition that powers evolution would have been exhausted long ago. The basic needs to feed and to breed coexist uneasily in the back forty of our brains, much too closely for comfort.

In other species, sexual competition and its expression through rituals of dominance are both obvious and unthreatening. We expect animals in the wild, from ruffed grouse to Siamese fighting fish, to put on displays of power as part of the mating process. We even accept extravagant expressions of sexual territoriality among higher primates, separated from ourselves by only a few strands of DNA, without moral judgment, but when it comes to ourselves, well, we're much too civilized for all that, aren't we?

Civilization certainly acts to channel and limit our Me-Tarzan/You-Jane impulses, but it does not make them go away. In fact, by repressing them it hydraulically compacts them into other forms of social, economic, and political competition, with results ranging from the admirable to the catastrophic. This is the process Freud called *sublimation*. What would happen if we were to experiment very, very carefully but directly with these impulses instead of brutally recasting them in their more socially acceptable manifestations? I don't think we would regress into our shaggy, club-wielding ancestors in a single generation. Neither do I believe for a moment that there would be no more war or that gender inequality would somehow vanish from the earth. However, I do think our sex lives would be more fun and more satisfying, and that is no small thing.

Let us for the moment, then, set aside inconclusive speculations about sociobiology, patriarchal indoctrination, unhealed childhood trauma, and original sin and accept that the desire to dominate a sex

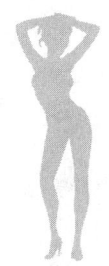

partner is normal and that its expression need not be destructive, abusive, or shameful. It is not a progressive addiction that leads to an uncontrollable lust for evermore extreme and dangerous practices; it's a hardwired component of our libidos over which we exercise individual responsibility. Now, let's assume we're talking about you.

Let's Talk This Over First— Thoroughly!

Have you ever wanted, even momentarily, to hold your partner down during sex and fuck him or her just as hard as you could? Have you ever had the desire to tease and hold back from your partner just long enough to make him or her ask for something before granting your permission? Have you ever contemplated asking your partner to "service" your needs first, before attending to his or her own? Do you get a rush when your lover swoons to your touch or get wet or hard when he or she is in your thrall? Do you desire to add ritual to your lovemaking, or props and costumes? Perhaps enacting scenarios addressing eternal themes of pursuit, capture, surrender, abandon, punishment, redemption, and force really gets your motor running.

Maybe you always want to remain on this side of the equation or perhaps you like to trade off who does what to whom every few minutes or every now and again. Perhaps you want to play this way every time or only every so often. If so, welcome to the wonderful world of power exchange, a heavily trafficked subset of sex play. For now, we'll address the dominant side of your inner world, saving the submissive person in the mirror for later introduction. Not everyone is wired for either kind of role playing, and, if you're not, you needn't worry that reading on out of curiosity will rearrange your basic circuitry. Power play isn't for everybody, and those who understand and enjoy it find plenty of company, so I'm not looking to make converts here.

The game of erotic domination and submission (D/s play for short) is predicated on the conscious and deliberate use of role structure and suspension of disbelief to bring fantasy to temporary life. For the duration of our theatrical reenactment, the dominant partner assumes the power to "compel" the submissive partner to behave as instructed within previously negotiated limits. The submissive partner permits him- or herself to be told what to do and when or for how long. Some D/s players prefer the term *top* for the person temporarily in charge and *bottom* for the receptive partner, but for the kinds of activities I'm describing here, which are more much more about role playing and feelings than about specific practices, the less technical terms *dominant* and *submissive* are more appropriate. For most occasional power players, the roles adopted for sex games have no applicability whatsoever outside the bedroom. While some dedicated D/s couples take on their "scene" identities as full-time lifestyles with varying degrees of success, it's best to assume that domination and submission stop at the bedroom door and that any attempt to exercise authority based on sex in other contexts violates the agreed conventions.

While discussions of sexual domination often devolve into loud arguments about gender, neither sex has a monopoly on power-play fantasies. Surprisingly while there are some gender-specific differences in the ways they tend to express themselves, as we'll discover, both men and women seem to find the basic pleasure of erotic power equally attractive. At various times, either sex might want to take charge of the sexual agenda, and either can do so with favorable results once certain basic concerns are addressed and resolved.

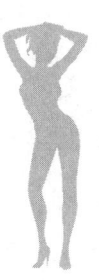

Sensual domination is a made-to-order pastime. It can be quite simple and basic or elaborate and complex, but in order for it to be ethical it must be founded on a few fundamental principles. If you are to play the dominant role in a sexual encounter, you must first negotiate the extent of your powers with your partner, accept without argument his or her limits, and observe those limits religiously. Without prior, informed, and enthusiastic consent, sexual domination is everything its critics deplore: abusive, exploitative, and potentially dangerous. It's also guaranteed to leave both players deeply unsatisfied.

One of the great delights of D/s sex is the emotional nakedness it affords its participants, but for that nakedness to be comfortable, it must be explored in a safe environment. That is why we negotiate limits and develop signals, sometimes called "safe words," to indicate when those limits have been reached. Nothing less than complete honesty is acceptable in the negotiating process. Neither of you should assent to anything you genuinely dislike simply to please the other. If, for instance, you establish in advance, as many D/s players do, that the word *yellow* will mean that whatever is going on is bordering on the unpleasant, the use of the word should immediately produce a return to the stop-and-talk phase. The word *red,* on the other hand, is a common signal used to put a full stop to all play activities until further notice. Once these boundaries have been drawn, they must be honored immediately and without argument.

In order to inhabit the sexually dominant role you play in your fantasies, you will first have to communicate what it is you want, hear and respect what your partner finds appealing or unappealing about your intentions, and arrive at a workable understanding. If, for instance, the movie in your head costumes you in a leather harness and boots while your naked partner licks his way up your legs before asking leave to eat your pussy, make those details clear in your explanation. Prepare to feel silly at first. No one is born knowing how to talk about these things, much less how to do them with suave self-assurance. If you have the right partner, your overriding positive regard for each other will get you through the more awkward revelations. If your partner has some specific embellishments of his or her own to add, you also enjoy the right to give or withhold consent. Some BDSM (short for bondage, discipline, sadism, and masochism) enthusiasts consider this "topping from the bottom," but I just call it good communication. You needn't feel that accepting suggestions compromises your dominant position or that you necessarily have to accede to them. My own dominant partner credits the creativity of previous submissive playmates for his mastery of a wide range of techniques and styles.

There is a possibility that you and your partner will prove incompatible when it comes to power play, and candid discussion may reveal this. Be prepared for the possibility of rejection. In the little scenario above, for example, the behavior I described was largely symbolic, involving no more than some costuming and a bit of dialogue. However, if you wish to add something like the use of a riding crop or flogger (a commonly used type of play whip with multiple, flat leather tails of varying weights), to induce a bit of sensation that falls short of actual pain, you may get a firm refusal. If you really want to use that whip aggressively, you might need to do so with someone else.

Depending on how powerful a component of your sexual character domination really is, you may have to adjust the notion of your "type" to include an individual whose submissive fantasies are as intense as your dominant fantasies. For occasional D/s players, accommodations are usually reached with relative ease. But for those to whom domi-

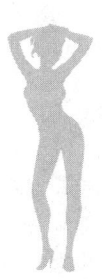

nance is a primary sexual turn-on, the prospects of long-term happiness with someone who finds the idea mildly appealing at best are not good. When you reveal your dominant strain to a partner, you run the risk of unearthing basic differences as well as common interests. This is all part of finding your sexual type, and sooner or later, the information will emerge. Talking it over first is the least risky way of eliciting that information.

Those whose primary sexual orientation involves regular activities in the realm of BDSM learn the hard way that dating or attempting to mate with nonkinky people just doesn't work. As it takes more than mere shared heterosexuality to make any couple a harmonious duet, out-of-the-ordinary sexual preferences also must dovetail for a relationship to succeed. A mismatch in this area will eventually unravel, just as it would between a swinger and a monogamous person trying to maintain a committed relationship.

Assuming that no deal breakers emerge, make a plan together and make it easy to start out with. Remember that role-play is foreplay, and at the end of whatever games you choose, the objective will be mutually volcanic sex. Those who somehow see domination as a substitute for fucking, sucking, munching, and other traditional activities pursuant to orgasmic release raise certain suspicions in me. Power play is something quite different from a power trip. I know denial and teasing are part of the dominant's arsenal of tricks and treats, but I'm assuming you're playing with a lover, and that is your primary role as well. Show me a dominant who feels compromised by giving head, and I'll show you a master or mistress soon to be unemployed. You and your partner may wish to put a time limit on the D/s portion of your engagement before proceeding to more conventional activities. Again, it's all about what you both want. For me, it's all about getting as excited as possible before getting down to the old-fashioned rock 'n' roll.

How Can Anybody Stand Up in These Boots?

Before you can take what you want, you first need to *know* what you want. This is actually the most challenging part of playing the dominant role effectively. Technique, mastery of terms and tackle, personal style, and all the other graces that mark the charismatic and capable "dom" can be acquired, but none will ring true with a partner unless and until you've figured out what turns you on about what you do.

Domination plays into my love of the dramatic, for instance. As an avid reader of historical literature and a high-school theater geek, I knew early on of my attraction to leather gloves, riding boots, women in corsets, and very, very high heels. Little did I know there were hundreds of thousands of others who shared the same attractions to certain objects of attire commonly called fetishes. I love the way I look outfitted as an equestrienne mistress or in a leather harness that accentuates my physique, and the structured interplay of a D/s "scene"—being called Ma'am or requiring my partner to ask permission for orgasm—allows me to perform for a particularly appreciative audience of one.

At the same time, my background as a nurse and sex educator naturally disposes me to play the authority figure in an affectionate context. One of my sources of dominant power lies in my willingness to provide tenderness and pleasure along with whatever rules I might enforce. I've found, logically enough, that the more fun I make our scenario for my partner, the more eagerly he or she will go along with my

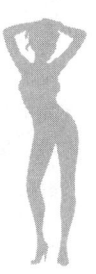

script. My partner's pleasure is the source of my power. I never hesitate to show my affection and appreciation for the gift of another's submission. If you've watched some "kinky" videos, you may have seen dominant performers barking at or berating submissives. I don't know about you, but if I wanted that, I'd try the Marines instead.

My greatest satisfaction in the dominant role comes from using my experience, my skills, and my imagination to take my partner to unexpected heights of sexual ecstasy, receiving grateful services in return. I wouldn't make such an exchange with someone for whom I felt no affection, much less for someone I held in contempt. My payoff is the power of pleasure and the feedback I get from using it responsibly and lovingly. I'd rather praise than criticize and please in order to be pleased.

But that's me. You and your partner must write your own script. In your conversations before the games begin, let it be known if you prefer to be a stern dominant, a playful dominant, a seductive dominant, or an affectionate dominant, or any combination thereof. Let your partner know what you want him or her to give you by way of satisfying your particular appetites. As we'll see when we explore sensual submission, the medium of exchange between "dominants" and "submissives" is shared stimulation. You must enjoy being pleased on the assumption that your partner enjoys pleasing you.

Once you and your playmate have figured out what it is about power play that turns you on, creating the atmospherics to stimulate those fantasies is a process of natural evolution. If, for example, you derive your satisfaction from exerting your power over some resistance, you and your partner might want to enact a scenario in which you are the demanding teacher who brings the naughty pupil into line. If you prefer a more direct route to sensual engagement, you may choose to be the master or mistress who commands his or her "slave" to provide anything from a massage to a bubble bath to oral sex as acts of servitude. If you have a taste for ritual, you may require a partner to dress in a certain manner, kneel to greet you, kiss your boots or shoes, or otherwise demonstrate submission through symbolic behavior. Tokens that reinforce role identity, such as a locking slave collar or a favorite pair of heels, help create the headspace in which power exchange becomes erotic.

Over a period of time, should you develop a strong interest in D/s play, you may find yourself acquiring a sophisticated skill set of BDSM techniques and the specially created "toys" used to employ them. However, the most important contribution you as a dominant bring to power play is your imagination.

Once the stage is set, it's the dominant's responsibility to keep the action moving toward the desired climax, to direct the "scene" from within. You're nominally in control (within the established rules), and you do most of the work: tying or untying, locking or unlocking, giving orders or receiving service, spanking or whipping. With practice, you'll be planning ahead three or four moves, keeping things safe and making sure your partner has as good a time as you. Far from being something you "do" to your submissive playmate, taking control in this way allows him or her to let go more completely and sink deeper into the experience. To encourage your partner to try challenging things, you must project a confident, welcoming, and relaxed attitude. The key element is trust, and it is empathy that makes trust possible. When you exchange power in a sexual context, you also exchange the ability to project yourselves into each other's roles and imagine how each of you experiences the parts you play. Without empathy, the whole paradigm breaks down, and neither party's needs are met.

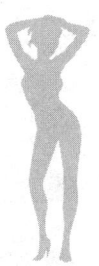

Keep in mind that consent is an ongoing process. You need to check in frequently, both physically and verbally, with your partner to be certain that he or she feels safe. Make certain that sense of safety is justified. You need to know what you're doing and know what you don't know how to do to be worthy of the trust placed in you. You may not unilaterally rewrite the script you've rehearsed halfway through. Don't try out a new toy or technique until its proper use has been shown to you, and preferably demonstrated on you, by someone with greater knowledge. Fortunately, a tradition of informal mentoring still prevails among D/s practitioners, and at any organized gathering, of which there are many every year throughout the country, you will find experts to teach you the proper use of a length of rope or a flogger.

I've found that complex techniques can be fun for a change of pace, but most D/s sex is simply sex as you already know it with the addition of role playing, and that is where I would invest my attention first before buying out the local tack shop or attending a seminar on Japanese-style rope suspensions. All that can come later if the interest is strong and mutual, but the emotional experience is what your submissive partner will remember and return to seek.

Creating Your Own Style

Consider the cover of a romance novel: the swashbuckling rogue and the swooning damsel. There is a reverse-gender archetype in a superheroine comic book: the exotically dressed amazon endowed with otherworldly powers and irresistible charm. Often, what we do in D/s play exaggerates and burlesques conventions regarding masculine and feminine ideals, bending, stretching, and supersizing them. Most of the time, we may be Edmond Dantes or Selena Kyles, but in the protected space of D/s play, we permit ourselves to be the Count of Monte Cristo or Catwoman. If you're to be effective in the dominant role with a member of the opposite sex, you need to build a style around the characters that exist in your imagination. Either a masculine or a feminine approach to domination should embody the most appealing aspects of those archetypes and as few as possible of the other kind.

The romantic image of the dominant man is strong, decisive, and powerful yet also protective and tender. The erotic dominatrix is proud, fearless, and willful but still vulnerable and charmingly seductive. Take these raw materials and shape them to reflect the character to which you want your partner to submit. Overbearing arrogance is the least appealing aspect of male domination and scolding condescension the female equivalent. These are bad places to start. Instead, try modeling your dominant persona on the playful, teasing, pleasing part of your affinity for your partner. You're not coming from an angry and disapproving place here, although you may need to feign stern judgment for a moment here and there. In this game, you're offering more rewards than punishments, with passionate sex the ultimate proof of your satisfaction. Comportment is all.

To dominate in a manly way, it helps to maintain good posture, move deliberately, and keep chatter to a minimum. Keep orders short and concise. You already enjoy the physical advantage, so your touch should be firm but not rough. I love having my hair pulled but hate having it yanked, so use your strength with sensitivity. In the submissive role, I'm glad to be told what to do, but I'll obey a voice of quiet authority far more eagerly than a barked command. I delight in being physically overpowered, but I don't expect to be tackled like a lineman. Modulate your approach. If your partner likes to play at resisting with

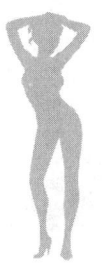

the ultimate goal of surrender, use only enough force to produce a panting acquiescence.

And give some thought to how you look. This is one place where men consistently fall short in the domination department, and it costs them more respect than they know. Women may not be as visual as men, but we do appreciate the efforts of a man who tries to look the part he's attempting to play. You can skip the Zorro outfit, but I've no intention of bowing down to kiss a ragged sneaker. How are you dressed when you feel most powerful? Are you most assertive in your boardroom suit, your motocross leathers, or your James Bond tuxedo? If you can't figure it out for yourself, go with simple, casual elegance in a dark color. Remember that a woman carries off theatrical flourishes more naturally than a man. We're accustomed to being looked at. If there is to be any kissing of shoes or boots, make them shiny, smooth, black, well-polished leather, please.

Always bear in mind that no level of technical accomplishment or inventory of impressive gear will take the place of the correct mind-set. We want to be dazzled by you, not by the array of gizmos and widgets in your secret closet.

A feminine style of domination may also involve specific abilities, but once again, the attitude you project is more important than what you actually do. If a man enjoys the advantage of physical strength, a woman can call upon her natural seductiveness. You already have something he wants, and in the dominant role, you determine how much of it he gets and when. Purring and slinking are far more effective than stomping and fuming. Touch him more boldly than you normally would. Take the initiative of undressing him or telling him to undress while you watch. Place his hands on your body where, when, and for exactly how long you desire. If you want your pussy eaten right now, this is one time you can tell him to get down on his knees and put his face between your thighs rather than hope he gets the idea on his own.

Learning to want, and then accept, service from our sex partners is a huge step for most women, since we're taught from an early age to be givers and not takers. If he really wants to please you in this way, however, who's "taking" anything except pleasure? Boldly stepping up to our own desire and passion opens the door for some amazing experiences. If a woman is supposed to be mysterious and alluring, take those notions to the extreme and tease him with your possibilities. It's not like you'll deny him his fondest wishes. Be aware of your movements. Slow and deliberate, confidently displaying yourself but keeping out of reach until you're ready to be touched is the approach that works most consistently.

Dominant women are often pictured in elaborate costumes of leather or latex, but lingerie and heels work just as well. You can go as wildly exotic with hair and makeup as you please, or stick to something flatteringly basic. There are many variations on the sexy and powerful look. I've done well with a trim-fitting suit and glasses. You may find yourself assuming the persona of nurse or schoolmistress, but the critical priority is to remain who you are underneath. Men don't want to be dominated by bitches any more than women want to be dominated by jerks. Man or woman, you are lover first and dominant second. Construct your image accordingly.

Making the Scene

Once you've agreed to play with domination and submission, what next? You may have read erotic stories about D/s play and have a general idea of what you want. Or you may only have fantasized about the concept in a general way. As a dominant, be direct about

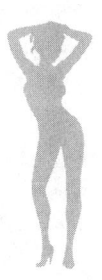

what you want. For example, how do you wish to be addressed? "Sir," "Master," "Ma'am," or "Mistress" are most common. I prefer "Ma'am" to "Mistress" unless my partner is English, in which case "Mistress" sounds delicious! If your submissive partner initiates the discussion and you have no clue what to do, let him or her explain how a particular fantasy works. He or she may want you to be forceful, imperious, demanding, loving, firm, or all of the above simultaneously. Stylized ways of speaking and acting help support the right mood while you fine-tune the details of your custom-built "session."

Try having your partner kneel in front of you, arms crossed at the small of the back, knees a bit open, posture tall and proud, as you circle him or her while making approving comments. Touching and caressing the head, a bit of hair pulling and letting your partner kiss the back of your hand are gestures that demonstrate both power and affection. I like to wear thin leather gloves (they feel delicious) and grasp my partner's lower jaw, pulling his or her face up to look at me. From that position, it's easy to push his or her head down to kiss my shoe.

It's also fun and easy to put my partner on his or her back, attach his or her wrist cuffs to the bed frame with some chain and carabineer clips, then put on a blindfold. Now my partner can't see what's coming next, reinforcing desired feelings of helplessness and anticipation. When your submissive is in this state, tease all over with a feather fan, velvet mitt, gently scratching nails, your own body, your mouth, leather floggers (great for dragging or striking), and other kinds of whips. Intersperse lots of genital contact to keep the heat rising. Drag your nipple close to his or her mouth or your crotch. Some people love the sensation of being nearly smothered in flesh. So guys, now's a good time to brush your cock and balls over your partner's face, pressing the bulb of your penis on her mouth and nose. For newly dominant women, the sensation of face sitting can be a potent rush. Having a submissive partner eagerly feel and taste you all over his or her face is a sensation I wish all women could experience at least once.

It's fun to sit on the couch, all done up in your favorite dominant look and have your submissive serve you in some way by bringing you a drink or a riding crop or a favorite paddle. Perhaps he or she has to kneel and present you with the desired item or to hold it in his or her teeth while crawling to you. It's very sexy to have your submissive stand in front of you for inspection of posture and costume. Ordering lewd display of the genitals can ratchet up the intensity, especially if your partner has shyness issues. Keep in mind that the more shy your partner is the more firm and approving you need to be. Your objective is to inspire pride in submission rather than shame.

If I've had my submissive bring me a striking device, such as a crop, cane, flogger, or whip, I like to get him or her very aroused before I use it. Not knowing when I'll strike is part of the fun. Some dominants may disagree, but I encourage masturbation during any kind of percussive play unless bondage is involved, as we'll discuss in our upcoming introduction to the joys of physical restraint. Any form of striking play is an obvious, physical assertion of dominance and, done properly, equally stimulating at either end of the equation. In the beginning of my kink education, when I was still wrapping my mind around some of this, it helped to think of it not as "mistreatment" (since there was no anger or abuse involved) so much as "stimulation application." It felt good to have my skin caressed and stimulated in this way, and I don't question what my body likes. As long as you never strike in anger, in the wrong place, or with the wrong instrument, it's safe to play with spanking, whipping, caning, flogging, etc. It's also an art form that needs instruction and practice to do well. A sudden, thoughtless

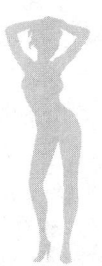

hip-wrap with a flogger, while more annoying than genuinely harmful, is a reliable mood breaker.

To more fully allow the submissive to go to "subspace," keep your order giving short and direct—"Give me your other end," "Crawl over there and bring me back the pillow," "Open your legs"—all spoken firmly but affectionately help set the proper tone. The same holds true for praise: "You're being very pleasing tonight." "You look good crawl-ing." "See how excited you get me?" Just a few words can evoke a much more elaborate fantasy in your partner's imagination.

When the kinky foreplay leads to its logical conclusion, you can take the active role and fuck your submissive, or you can order your submis-sive to fuck you. Who's on top doesn't necessarily determine who's in charge. To sit in your favorite chair while your partner gives you a great lap dance (the one without clothes) makes you feel powerful and your other half desirable, but so does being on top and having your way with him or her. You can tell your partner to lie still while you set the pace, or be still yourself and have him or her do the work. Holding your part-ner's hands above his or her head, or attaching them with chains, clips, or rope is, perhaps, the most literal way of asserting sexual dominance. The use of eye contact to stay connected also increases your power.

It's always good to intersperse conventional intercourse with D/s play, such as pausing for more oral service from your partner, spanking, flogging, or paddling between positions, or sending your "slave" to fetch something just for the pleasure of watching an appealingly naked form move about the room. You can masturbate yourself while telling your submissive to do the same. Putting on a good show for a dominant part-ner is a source of real satisfaction to many submissive players.

If I'm dominating a multiorgasmic partner, I make sure he or she has all the orgasms he or she can stand before I have my usual one. If my partner is singly orgasmic, I'll draw out the plateau phase for as long as humanly possible before pushing him or her over the edge.

When we've both had our fill, I like to spend as much time in the afterglow as we can. We can be silent, basking in the endorphins engendered by a rip-roaring "sesh," or verbally replay the highlights. It's also very important to process the complex mixture of emotions stirred by such a powerful experience, at least while you're still getting to know each other's inner workings. When my dominant partner and I were new to D/s play together, we talked a lot after each encounter. Now, we hardly need to at all, except for giving each other a happily exhausted high five. At the end, at the beginning, and all the way through, communication is the most important guarantee of a mutually satisfying D/s experience.

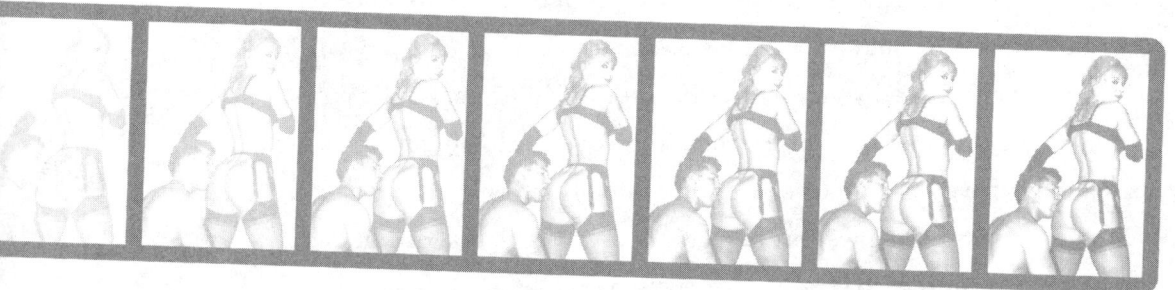

Top Tips

1 · *Give the right orders.* It's not that hard to get people to do things they don't want to do. That happens at the office every day. The trick lies in figuring out what people really do want to do and giving them permission to enjoy it.

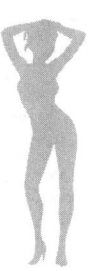

2 • *Keep it light.* This is meant to be fun. Don't be afraid to flirt, show affection, give approval, and have a laugh or two. Since you have no real authority in your fantasy world, you needn't worry about undermining it.

3 • *What you say is as important as what you do.* People are less fragile physically and more fragile emotionally than you might suppose. A tiny bruise is less a concern than hurt feelings.

4 • *Let your dark side show.* If you've found your way to the right partner, he or she probably already knows more about your perverse urges than you think, and that's exactly what's wanted out of you.

5 • *Keep the sex happening at all times.* Whether giving a spanking or engaging in some light bondage play, stop frequently to mix in plenty of direct stimulation. Remember, it's all foreplay.

6 • *Be creative.* Ritualized sex play can get repetitive and monotonous. Change it up with different times, places, costumes, and situations.

7 • *Keep learning.* Whether or not you want to be the kind of dom who knows every esoteric technique in the vast lore of BDSM, the more you know about how others play, the more your own imagination will be inspired.

8 • *Take a hint.* Your submissive partner's inner desires are your best allies in making the D/s experience pleasurable for both of you, but first you need to know what they are, even if the information takes a little time and coaxing to emerge.

DOMINANT DOWNERS

1 • *Don't take yourself too seriously.* It's easier than you can imagine for domination to descend into self-parody.

2 • *Forget about trying to prove how great you are at this game.* The only proof of that is the mutual satisfaction you and your partner will share.

3 • *It's not about who has the biggest toy bag.* Don't turn your D/s play into just another expensive hobby and excuse to show off flashy status symbols.

4 • *Never try anything on anyone else that you haven't experienced yourself.*

5 • *Forget the whole idea of punishment as anything but an excuse to give your partner what he or she really wants anyway.* If you're genuinely angry about something, you shouldn't play until you're over it. That way lies abuse.

6 • *Your powers end at the bedroom door.* Just because your lover wants to be your slave in bed doesn't mean you get your laundry done for free.

7 • *No barking, scolding, woofing, huffing, stomping, or other inauthentic display of pique.* This is a particular failing of female dominants wobbly in their stilettos and trying too hard.

8 • *Don't push.* If you meet strong resistance to a particular demand, drop it for good. That doesn't mean try it again five minutes later to see if your partner's had a change of heart.

Chapter 16

SENSUAL SUBMISSION: GIVING IT UP FOR LOVE

f taking the submissive role in bed is your preference, prepare to defend your choice. Expect others to have all sorts of opinions and judgments about it, however uninformed. In our highly competitive society, with its unrelenting emphasis on the need to be in control at all times, submissive sexuality remains largely closeted, and no wonder. Its stereotypical portrayal in popular culture and the relentless negativity to which it has been subjected by political ideologues and rigid psychiatric professionals have given it a whole list of bad names. If dominants have been wrongly labeled abusive, antisocial, and misogynistic, sexual submissives have been told they're weak, pathetic, self-hating, brainwashed traitors to their respective genders and victims of a progressive addiction that can lead only to their doom.

I was surprised to find how many of these misconceptions I harbored myself, and I'm supposed to be open-minded!

What do I know now about sexual submission that I didn't know ten years ago? First and foremost I've learned that *submit* is a verb, indicating an action taken or a choice made. Consensual submission is not a form of self-abnegation; it's the opposite. It takes a confident individual to willingly surrender the initiative, even temporarily, especially in the face of social hostility. To borrow the declaration of a female friend of mine, "As a modern, liberated woman, I've had to learn to demand to be controlled." It's a radical notion, and I didn't embrace it easily. A product of the feminist thinking of my own time to some degree, I struggled to reconcile my beliefs about the importance of freedom and equality with my sexual fantasies of yielding to a distinctly masculine power. I didn't realize just how much company I had out there until I began to discuss openly my own struggle with the allure of submission, only to find that a large proportion of my generation of women felt equally conflicted about the contradictions between what they wanted in bed and what they wanted in life.

A submissive doesn't submit to the other person as much as he or she submits to the pleasure of the experience while making it clear that taking unfair advantage of his or her sexual nature will not be tolerated. A desire to submit in the bedroom says exactly nothing about who we are or what we expect anyplace else. I've known many sexually submissive men and women, and I would characterize them overall as assertive personalities and independent thinkers who don't believe their sexual fantasies should be subject to plebiscite. As with those who generally play in the dominant role, the ultimate goal of the sensual submissive is to cross wire the powerful currents of aggression and sexual desire to generate high-voltage sex of the more familiar kind (what

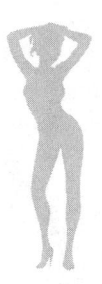

kinky people call "vanilla" fucking and sucking), with the dynamo dialed up by role-playing activities that combine the two.

Both genders get mixed messages concerning submission. For much of human history women have been told to submit in both the public and private spheres. We've been exhorted to submit to the authority of village elders, shamans, priests, the church, our fathers, uncles, brothers, husbands, and sons, and to the judgment of our own kind regarding what is considered respectable. All of this has been for our own good, of course, in accordance with "natural" law. Women have borne and, in many parts of the world, continue to bear, untold suffering in the name of this particular conception of femininity right up to the present day.

More recently, at least in Western culture, women have been told the opposite. Now we can (and must!) take charge, both in the world at large and in the bedroom. If we don't adhere to the party line in every particular, we're pitiful victims, enablers, or self-serving collaborators with the enemy gender. This has engendered shame and confusion among women who do wish to be submissive in bed and now feel somehow defective for their own authentic preferences. I fail to see how this is an improvement over being denied our right to seek any other form of personal satisfaction.

Men have been equally burdened with crushing expectations of how their identities should be properly defined. They've been told since time immemorial that they must be in command under all circumstances and to want anything else, no matter what, no matter where, is to be weak and effeminate. Over the past one hundred years or so they've been ordered to reverse course, at least in our society. Now they're told if they do desire to rule in bed, they're acting under the sway of patriarchal conditioning or testosterone poisoning. Men are currently instructed to figuratively castrate themselves on the altar of political correctness, the consequences to their sex lives and those of their partners be damned.

One might suppose that this change in popular dogma would create an earthly paradise for submissive men, but such is hardly the case. We encourage men to open up to their true feelings and then disrespect and denigrate them when they do. While old definitions of masculinity have come under attack, however warranted, there has been no new model showing how a man might be different and still be considered masculine to replace them. The expectations of other men haven't necessarily evolved in a more accepting manner. An individual woman may be thrilled that her husband or lover wants to be sexually submissive, but he won't be able to share that part of himself with his male friends. If one set of inaccurate and destructive stereotypes of femininity has replaced another, confusion reigns where progressive role models for men are concerned. Are they supposed to be Mr. Mom or Rambo or some indefinable combination of both?

Male submission is still tainted with such shame that a specialized subset of discreet professional dominatrixes has evolved to service it commercially. Whatever the particulars (mommy, nurse, teacher, boss, femme fatale), "pro doms" enact their clients' fantasies of female authority at an hourly rate. Their trade flourishes precisely because so few women are comfortable taking control in bed or even find the idea appealing enough to attempt (though more might if they understood the options better). Some submissive men long to incorporate their sexuality into romantic relationships while others prefer to keep the two separate, but neither group finds it easy to get all their needs met in one place.

In an atmosphere of confusion and conflict over definitions of "appropriate" masculine and feminine behavior, either a man or a woman, however open-minded regarding other forms of sexual expression, may

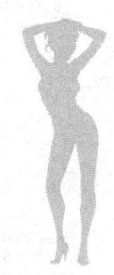

feel like a traitor to his or her gender by acting out fantasies of erotic submission. This response is understandable but groundless. Behaving contrary to gender stereotypes, new or old, by what you do in bed doesn't betray the other 3 billion people worldwide who share an XX or XY chromosome with you. The only person to whom you'll be untrue if you don't explore this side of yourself if you want to, or try to make yourself do so if you don't, is you. Regardless of what society tells you about what's right for your gender, you'll ultimately have to form an identity for yourself. Even choosing not to do so constitutes a decision and generally not the one that will lead to the greatest personal satisfaction.

The reality of sexual submission is very different from its portrayal in popular culture, whether for laughs, thrills, shock, terror, or propaganda. It's not about pain, and it does not replace conventional sexual intercourse. It is pleasure seeking through erotic surrender. Sexual submissives have opinions, likes, and dislikes; things they'll do and things they won't. Sexual submission is not an indicator of low self-esteem or a need/desire to be abused or taken advantage of. It's not women's "natural" place or a man's "unnatural" one. Submissives are not the inferiors of their dominant partners. Rather, they are equals in this dance of seduction deeply rooted in human experience, each needing the other to complete the ceremony. A favorite lover reminds me that "there's no pride or challenge in dominating a weak person. I'd rather have a tiger at the end of my leash than a house cat."

Why Submission?

Erotic submission is a contract between two equals, an expression of trust, an effective avenue to arousal, and a potent means of self-expression. To let another person into your heart and mind, to give him or her the "keys to the kingdom," and to trust that this person will not abuse that gift can create sexual magic. For some lucky individuals, slipping into a submissive headspace is as easy as breathing; for others, the longing for surrender is a source of endless inner conflict that must be overcome by dint of concentrated effort. Domination and submission are body-based activities that also require the active participation of the imagination. I can submit only for as long as my partner plays my body properly, and only a dominant who learns to read the emotional cues of a submissive lover will engender the trust he or she needs to play the dominant part effectively.

Sexual submission feels a lot different than it looks. I used to see pictures of women in collars and leashes and wonder why any self-respecting person would identify herself as a sex slave. The idea of a person crawling on hands and knees to kiss a boot or high-heeled shoe made me scratch my head in wonder. Now, having done these things myself, I have some answers. To an uninformed outsider, the collar and leash might seem to signify degradation or dehumanization, but the person wearing them feels cherished, like a prized possession, special to the person holding the other end, secure in the agreed boundaries of a role, and safe in the affections of his or her partner. By the nature of the D/s relationship, such props are imbued with a special meaning. When the collar and leash are on, the submissive must behave in a certain way, yes, but so must the dominant. Much D/s behavior is symbolic in this way, and these symbols liberate our fantasies even as they constrain our physical selves.

Crawling to kiss the boot or shoe is an act of devotional worship, a moment of heightened emotion for both players. As the crawling person, I like to make sure my form is perfect, my posture composed and confidant: an iconic image for the dominant to admire. In the kissing of

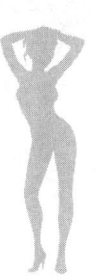

a boot or shoe, I express respect for the dominant's position as well as my own desire for his or her attentions and affection. It's a moment of freedom, as I inflect that kiss with my feelings for the person to whom I give myself as a gift, even if only temporarily. No matter what the activity, it's the emotion with which it's invested that matters.

A knowing and effective dominant partner's attention will focus sharply on you and your body's responses. In that way, the exchange of feeling within the constraints of ritual is very romantic, as when you were first dating and new to each other. Submission renders you at once attainable and inscrutable. As you invent your "character" in role, there can always be more to know about you. I enjoy erotic submission because it offers me the perfect stage upon which to refine the courtesanlike skills of sexual service, to show myself off as the polished instrument of pleasure I've trained myself to become.

If this attitude seems to welcome the dreaded objectification about which we're so relentlessly belabored about the head and ears, it's based on the understanding that such objectification is transient and by my own choice. When the game is over, I'll go back to being my independent and often contrary self, more confident and determined than ever. When I'm perfecting my posture, or my crawling, or my kneeling, or my serving of wine, I invest each movement with my own will to connect through the shared experiences of power and pleasure. In this way, submission is like a martial art: movement and meditation toward a purposeful objective. I'm fully aware of my ass and how it looks, of my pussy and how it's wet, of my mouth and how it wants to taste my partner's cock. And I'm equally sure he is tuned to the same frequency because the signal strength between us is so cracklingly apparent.

You know how good it felt when you were younger to master a new skill: driving, balancing a checkbook, or cooking a full dinner without mishap? The learning curve of erotic submission offers some of the same satisfactions. There's the blow job you gave when you were new to oral sex; there's the blow job you give now; and then there's the blow job you give with bells, whistles, cute costume, and perfect positioning, all without seeming to break a sweat. It requires more resourcefulness than you think to be able to juggle your own responses and behavior and how you communicate them within your self-imposed limits as well as his or her responses. Clearly, the submissive role is anything but passive. Done for the right reasons and with the right person, sexual service provides a means to be creative, express your love and devotion in a truly personal way, and earn yourself the reward of what may well be some of the hottest bonking in your life.

With the right person at the right time and for the right motives, erotic submission is sublime, romantic, intoxicating, energetic, challenging, satisfying, and authentic. Under the wrong conditions, it can be dangerous, foolish, awkward, crazy, stupid, and unwise. I have observed D/s situations that truly lived down to popular expectations, and it is your responsibility as a sensible, self-respecting individual to avoid them. Embrace what makes you wet or hard and reject what makes you dry or deflated. Follow your body's honest responses, and you'll find your proper location on the D/s continuum. And make sure you don't abandon your good judgment along the way. You're playing with potent forces of nature here, and it's your obligation to do so consciously and responsibly.

Submission Skill Sets

There are many methods submissive players use to get into "subspace," that rarified place of deep surrender and unification where they respond easily and naturally, and feel fully connected to

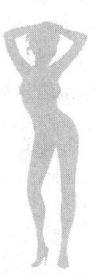

their partners. These methods include ritual forms of address, the creative use of costumes and props, acts of erotic servitude, and behaviors that best express the will to surrender.

Dominants can't read minds and shouldn't be expected to. If we, as submissives, want positive experiences, we must communicate our needs and limits clearly and without embarrassment. Before you can let go as you desire, your dominant must know all he or she can about your preferences, your positive and negative triggers (words or deeds), your greatest turn-ons and biggest turnoffs as well as any physical limitations that would get in the way of certain postures or behaviors (bum knee, sciatica, etc.). Any hard limits on behavior or language must be communicated clearly. Be specific. If covering your mouth is fine but not your nose and mouth together, say so. Perhaps no aspect of the submissive skill set is as challenging as communicating sensitive information without breaking your role or spoiling the mood.

Remember that anyone worth submitting to wants your creative input to improve the experience for both of you. He or she will feel more secure if you express yourself clearly and therefore inhabit the dominant role with greater confidence. This is especially important if your dominant partner still struggles to overcome PC bullshit about D/s sex and feels residual guilt about "treating you this way." Your very lack of embarrassment and ambivalence helps him or her overcome stubborn, internal resistance to assuming command. After all, you may be the first proud, confidant submissive he or she has ever met.

Even after the game has begun, there are many ways in which you can telegraph desires without using words, breaking character, or spoiling the moment. Like Morse code, each movement or body position conveys a meaning that a well-chosen dominant partner will interpret to your mutual benefit. Kneeling with hands behind you or with fingers laced behind your neck signals your availability. Not looking your partner in the eye without permission or invitation suggests a willingness to cede the initiative. Showing off your ass is both an invitation and a challenge. Wiggling it back and forth means it wants attention, whereas holding your butt cheeks open says, "I'm in an anal mood." Holding your legs open while touching yourself signals your rising heat. Fucking yourself with a toy for your partner's entertainment demonstrates both a sincere desire to please and an enthusiasm for "naughty behavior" if the opportunity presents itself. What makes these acts so arousing is their explicit expression of both a will to yield and a powerful sexual intent. A sex slave is expected to be sexual and thus liberated from shame. While your nominal obligation is to the satisfaction of your dominant partner, your unspoken objective is to get some for yourself whenever and wherever possible.

Language is used to reinforce the power dynamic, role structure, and hierarchy. The actual forms of address aren't as important as their consistent use. When you do speak, you can be as direct as you have to: "I like to be held down while you fuck me," "I really love it when you pull my hair and make me go down on you," "I need to be spanked and teased while you tell me how naughty I've been," "Please, Sir, may I come/pee/touch myself?" and "Please, Ma'am, may I eat your pussy?" are all appropriate ways of expressing your wants and feelings. If I want to wear a particular article of clothing or behave in a particular way during our play, I'll ask if Sir would like to see me in a hood/corset/ballet boots. This lets him know that I'm interested in a particular activity within the role structure. Any partner who doesn't welcome this subtle give-and-take as part of the fun of D/s play needs to do more homework. When first learning to play this way, I could hardly refrain from laughing at how odd it felt, and how shy I was, at speaking in such a stilted,

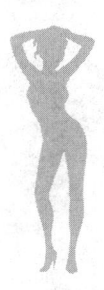

"unnatural" manner. As I became more experienced, the shyness abated, leaving only confidence in my ability to hold my own in this game.

A self-realized submissive is proud of his or her abilities and knows the value of the gift being offered. His or her movements reflect a reaching for excellence. Good submissives are a little like ballet dancers: Every motion, no matter how small, is imbued with meaning and purpose. Stand tall, chin straight, eyes modestly downcast, hands bent at the elbows and folded behind the small of the back. Ready, poised to go in any direction. Being still like this helps your concentration, especially if, like me, you have a lot of internal chatter to silence for sex to achieve its full potential. A good submissive is centered, neither drifting away in boredom nor anticipating what the dominant might want next. When moving, a good submissive is conscious of being watched, knowing that the dominant appreciates every angle, every fluid motion. Knowing you're being watched definitely makes you walk, crawl, or pour a glass of wine more consciously. We're all insecure about our bodies. Learning to enjoy visual appreciation is a form of liberation in itself.

The most common honorifics for dominants are "Master," "Mistress," "Sir," and "Ma'am." You and your partner get to choose which, if any, to use or to come up with your own. Actual "punishment" has no constructive use in consensual D/s play, but the notion of playfully applied disciplinary measures can serve as useful reminders until proper form becomes second nature. Knowing I liked the drama of it, my dominant partner would give me a little slap on the face when I neglected to add "Sir" in an answer to a direct question: "Is that too tight?" "No." "No, what?" (little slap) "No, Sir." "Good girl." (kiss) The tone should be nothing except flirtatious or loving, no matter how harsh the vocabulary, since this is a pleasure game, not a power trip. As a submissive, with prenegotiated limits, you have every right to respectful treatment, even when you "misbehave."

It's vitally important that, during a D/s session, "punishment" is *never* motivated by anger or by the desire to inflict actual pain. Real pain and punishment have little to do with consensual D/s play, even if the participants consider themselves "sadistic" or "masochistic." Obviously, though a physical sensation can be extremely powerful and possibly unpleasant in a different context, if its purpose is ultimately to produce pleasure, it can't really be considered painful. As a submissive, you may be deliberately disobedient at times for the fun of it, and you can and should expect your dominant partner to present you with difficult challenges from time to time in order to keep things exciting, but motive and context are everything, and a mutual desire to please is the foundation of all responsible D/s play. One skill every submissive should cultivate is the ability to speak up when this principle is violated.

D/s is a game between lovers and as such is no place for passive/aggressive acting out. Punishments are part of play, meted out both for fun and for reinforcement of compliance with the agreed-upon rules, such as one stroke with the paddle for every minute a submissive is late, or a couple of minutes spent as a human footstool for forgetting to use the proper honorific. The submissive can even give the dominant ideas as to good ways to "correct" him or her for the lapses that inevitably occur. To honor the spirit of the game, though, the suggestions should be at least a bit challenging. You can always make a dominant smile by requesting a couple of extra spanks for whatever you've done wrong. It's a playful demonstration of your eagerness to please and helps you get past any real embarrassment you may feel over whatever mistake you've made.

Since D/s play is a form of erotic theater, costumes can be very helpful in setting the stage and making the fantasy real. Just as a dom-

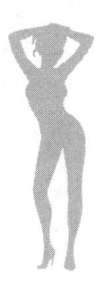

inant might use items of attire to get in the right mood (boots, gloves, masks, etc.), there are totems a submissive can adopt to heighten the effect. You need enough clothing to symbolize your status but not so much as to obstruct its enjoyment.

The most common item is the slave collar. In this usage, *slave* is understood to mean "love slave," a voluntary, temporary status with terms negotiated between the players. The collar marks a submissive as special, "owned," wanted, desired, valued, and the "property" of the dominant for the duration of playtime. This item can be an actual collar, either custom-made or purchased from a pet store, sex shop, or BDSM gear supplier. It can also be something simple and symbolic, like a special necklace or a ribbon. One woman I know telegraphs her desire for a D/s session by wearing a pretty choker her boyfriend gave her. That way, she can play the Coy Thing and he can still be confident that she will accept his advances. A couple can create a ritual for the putting on and taking off of the collar. One dominant I know always kisses the back of his submissive's neck before locking it on. This small gesture is a reminder of the romantic nature of what is to come, as if he's putting on a diamond necklace. A male submissive can also wear a collar, of course, generally something leather and a bit heavier and more macho. Men are usually taller than women, so he can present her with the collar before kneeling to accept it.

Another wardrobe item popular among submissive women is a pair of the highest, sexiest heels that she can walk or stand in and that never go outside or serve any other purpose. By keeping them unscathed, she's always as pretty as a picture, a perfect "love doll." An added benefit of the very-high-heeled shoe is that it is a form of bondage that requires no rope at all, since she can't walk very far or fast in them and they reinforce her temporary helplessness.

Other clothing items that submissives adopt include stockings and garters, leather body harnesses, studded jock straps, long gloves, ankle and wrist cuffs, and corsets. Full nudity is also a frequent preference of both dominants and submissives, as nothing else so complete conveys the impression of total vulnerability. All of these costume approaches use fetishistic cues to convey a certain mood, and like every other element of a satisfying encounter, they're subject to negotiation. If he really wants you to wear a corset but you're too uncomfortable to fuck in it, he may have to settle for a light waist cincher. If joint problems prohibit walking in those skyscraper heels, perhaps you'll just have to crawl instead or lie on your back and wave them in the air. And a man who feels ridiculous in a leather harness isn't going to give you his best sexual performance, so you may have to take him in the raw.

Sexual servitude is an enduring theme in D/s play. The services to be rendered are up to the two of you to devise. The more personally meaningful they are the better. It's important to imbue the action with the right attitude, usually one of gratitude, pleasure, reverence, and a willingness to serve. A submissive should never "just put up with" something or go through the motions, though. A submissive's heart being in the right place is important to the successful outcome of a session. Serving food or drinks in special dishes or glasses or feeding favorite treats by hand are love-service gestures. Being available to perform oral sex while fully or partially clothed without the expectation of immediate reciprocation demonstrates a selfless wish to please. Washing your partner's back in the tub, brushing his or her hair, shaving his or her genitals, and/or helping your dominant to dress are classic love-slave services. Laying out whatever toys or props are to be used during play and creating the proper environment with mood lighting,

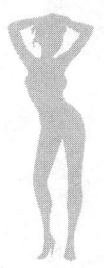

music, candles, etc., are common submissive duties. Cleaning up after play is in the same category.

At the risk of generalizing from anecdotal experience, I find male submissives more disposed toward practical labors—running errands, fixing things around the house, etc.—whereas female submissives tend toward directly sexual or at least domestic acts of servitude, like waiting, attired only in apron and heels, to offer a drink to her husband on returning from work, for example. It's really the sentiment rather than the action that matters. The expression of the desire to please is the submissive's most potent tool of seduction.

In my vision of sexual submission, which is by no means the only one, all of these activities are preliminary to a volcanic sexual consummation. The erotic tension implicit in the game of D/s is released at the moment of actual penetration, when your offer is accepted in a forceful and unambiguous way. The combined, determined attentions of the two of you create the atmosphere of an idealized (if perverse) wedding night. All the foreplay, teasing, serving, showing off, bondage, and/or spanking play, along with whatever little touches you invent between you, intensify the physical sensations of intercourse to the point of intoxicating euphoria. All the care and consideration you put into the preliminaries are rewarded with a level of passionate response from both of you that's worth every moment of effort and forethought you're invested. It's important to keep the game going during sex and not revert to your regular selves like Cinderella's pumpkin coach. Don't dispense with the more formal ways of speaking once the fucking starts, or forget that you're still a fascinating sex creature. The longer you can sustain the mood, the higher the temperature will rise.

Writing Your Own Script

Every submissive player eventually develops a favorite "scene" persona, a projected image that helps him or her maintain a state of aroused surrender. Sometimes the stylistic touches are very subtle; other times, quite dramatic. All help create contexts for the type of play that suits a particular couple's fantasies. There are some basic types, but I'm sure you'll figure out your own: the Brat, the Good Girl/Boy, the Stoic, the Complainer, the Slut, the Innocent, and the Service Slave are popular standards. The Brat mildly misbehaves to elicit a stern response. The Stoic might prefer to be pushed to a physical limit in order to feel stripped of inhibitions. To heighten the dramatic atmosphere the Complainer likes to fuss, moan, and whine while performing the required tasks or during the earned punishment. The Slut might have to show off his or her wares or masturbate for a partner's amusement so any loss of modesty can be attributed to the requirements of the role. The Innocent might have to be told how to do every little thing, milking each for maximum attention value. The Service Slave gets his or her thrill from vicariously enjoying a partner's pleasure. As you can see, the submissive is never without agency, even if its expression is indirect.

Likewise, with a steady playmate, you'll develop your own menu of favorite activities and preferences as to when and how to organize them. If you're already interested in or familiar with D/s play you've probably found other sources of information by now. If not, you'll discover a world of books, websites, and organizations of similarly inclined adventurers from whom you can learn how D/s or BDSM play can be polished for the greatest satisfaction. Like swinging, D/s play is a social as well as individual activity, with many local, state, and national groups offering classes and other educational services. When you find

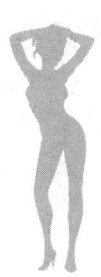

your way to the community, there will be people you like and people you don't; ethical, upright citizens and out-and-out jerks; friendly couples and aloof ones. The territory here is uncharted for you and your partner, making it extra important to be scrupulous in making rules and charting courses. Some people combine swinging with D/s play and some don't. Either way, it won't hurt to consult our earlier discussion of swinging for reminders on proper etiquette and cautions regarding any kind of intimate relations in group settings. Kinksters have special rules of their own, but certain basics regarding honesty and respect for the boundaries of others apply in both communities.

The most important education in the ways of D/s sex play is that which you give each other through the course of your private experimentation. Thousands of couples already engage in some kind of D/s activity without formally acknowledging it. If you've ever deliberately "provoked" your partner into chasing you, catching you, and throwing you down on the bed, that's D/s energy at work. If a playful spanking adds to the enjoyment of such a game, you may be further along than you thought. If you've ever offered yourself up with a ribbon around your neck for extra-special oral service on your lover's birthday, you've got the basic idea of sensual service somewhere in your head.

If you hope to make such activities more regular and more formal, you'll need to be fearlessly candid about the specifics. If you want to play on the submissive side of the equation, you'll require the full and enthusiastic participation of a dominant partner who you trust and respect in deciding how big a part to assign this preference in the overall construction of your relationship. One of you may find just the great costumes and bit of scripted dialogue enough of a turn-on, while the other wants the whole range of ritualistic behavior that goes along with the outfits, and that may or may not be negotiable. Some combinations work much better than others. A dom and a sub of similar predispositions balance the scales best, but two people who like to switch can reach a good understanding, sometimes with the benefit of a kitchen timer or a coin to flip to determine who does what to whom first or for how long. Two doms or two subs have a less of a chance of working out something mutually beneficial, no matter how much they may like each other or what other compatibilities they may enjoy.

An early relationship of mine foundered on that very shoal. I had no understanding of D/s dynamics or where on the continuum I fell, and neither did he. I didn't understand what I now realize was his essential submissiveness and found it confusing at the time when I was young and inexperienced. I would know what to do with it now, of course, but I also know that I don't want a submissive as my primary mate. If a person really needs to be in one role or the other to fully enjoy a sexual experience, nothing else can substitute. If a person has no taste or affinity for it, nothing can change that, either. You cannot make your partner into your dominant if he or she doesn't want to go there. Too many of my submissive friends, frustrated by the lack of caring, competent doms out there, have chosen to involve themselves with otherwise perfectly fine individuals who were vanilla to the core, hoping to somehow bring them around. You can't make a person want, or like, D/s sex no matter how "perfect" he or she might be in every other way.

Some submissives delude themselves that, because they're offering their bodies and their affections so generously, no sane person could refuse them. And the novelty of such an approach may stir some passing interest in an otherwise non-D/s-oriented person who finds him or her attractive for other reasons, but sooner or later the requirements of the dominant role will wear out that passing appeal, often with bitter consequences. If you discover that the desire for erotic submission is an in-

tegral part of your sexual identity, you owe it to yourself and others to seek out or accept only those potential mates with similar enthusiasms. This will naturally narrow your choice of candidates to a frustrating degree and you may need considerable patience to hold out for what you really need, but no other course of action is wise or humane. Since you can't change your fundamental sexual orientation any more than you could your fingerprints, you'll find happiness only with someone who wants you as who and what you are. The first person who has to fully accept and embrace your submissive nature, if that's truly what you're about, is you. That will be the hardest part. Once you're at ease with this aspect of your character, you'll tend to attract others of a similar sexual type.

Once again, just as dominant personalities must, you may need to look outside the conventions of your fantasies about the "perfect" mate for you and consider more unconventional choices. I have a good friend—young, beautiful, smart, gifted, and ambitious but very conservative in her taste in men—who has had nothing but bad luck trying to square her broader expectations of a mate with her powerful hunger for the satisfactions of sexual submission. She keeps trying to shape one decent, square vanilla guy after another into her dream dominant and keeps ending up alone and frustrated. So she will remain until she begins to cast her net a bit wider.

When it came to writing the book of our own marriage, my current husband and I had to discard some elements of our earlier personal narratives. He had always imagined himself mated to a woman who identified herself as much by her submission as he does by his dominance. I had written my own story primarily around my calling as a performer and a sex educator with the delivery of a message about sexual liberation as my primary mission. In a very real sense, we're both dominantly inclined, though fortunately in significantly different ways. Owing to our shared misfortunes from attempting to make our private lives conform too closely to our public representations of them, we've been able to form a bond that transcends our differences. I can now accept my own need for submission just as he can accept its limits. In this way, it enhances our erotic lives together without defining them.

As a submissive, you can reasonably be expected to be pleasing and seductive but not to flash in public, to give a few minutes of oral sex to start the day but not if you're under the weather, to get the play space ready ahead of time but not to know automatically what gear should be laid out, to have a concern for a dominant partner's wishes but not to overlook your own needs. Some dominants enjoy the power of sharing a submissive partner's attention with a friend. If you like the idea and the friend, you can satisfy to such a request, but your compliance can never be required.

Ultimately, though a dominant may propose, it is up to a submissive to accept or decline. Both set their erotic agenda. With that precept clearly in mind, there is much enjoyment to be had and little risk involved in allowing yourself the privilege of surrender for a set period of time. In a world where competition rules so much of our daily lives, where we must be on our guard against so many potential risks, a safe

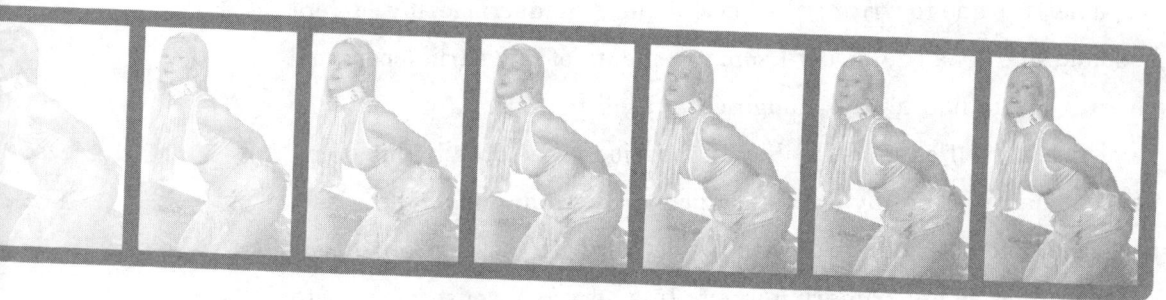

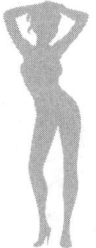

space in which to know ourselves through willed surrender is a lovely luxury. The choice to find that space is entirely your own and none of anyone else's concern.

SECRETS OF SUBMISSION

1 · *Be good but not perfect.* Your human self with its human failings is the source of your allure.

2 · *Cultivate the arts of giving pleasure as ends in themselves.* You'll get your best rewards by seeking to please rather than to be pleased.

3 · *Keep it light.* A naughty sense of humor helps maintain a properly playful tone.

4 · *Demonstrate your respect by presenting yourself at your most appealing,* based on what your dominant partner has expressed in the way of likes and dislikes.

5 · *Be aware of your body language.* Don't be afraid to let your enjoyment show.

6 · *Let your creativity inspire your partner.* If you have a hot submissive fantasy you'd like to act out, find a respectful way to share it.

7 · *Allow yourself to be affectionate in your submission.* Dominants need appreciation too.

8 · *Take pride in what you do.* Whether it's giving head or administering an erotic massage, you should appreciate yourself as you expect to be appreciated.

9. *· Take good care of the equipment.* A gel-filled pad for the knees is a must.

Sub Sinkers

1 • *Don't lie.* Never say you like what you hate or hate what you like. You owe your partner the truth about your tastes and desires.

2 • *Avoid breaking role,* even when you need to express dissatisfaction. Raise whatever concerns you may have in a respectful manner.

3 • *Never recriminate after the fact.* If something happens in a D/s situation that crosses your boundaries, speak up at the time.

4 • *Using your submissive charms, or withholding them, to secure nonsexual rewards is a violation of trust* that shouldn't be tolerated and won't be for long by anyone worth having.

5 • *There are errors in any game.* Don't judge your partner's too harshly, lest yours be judged in the same light. You'll make them, I promise.

6 • *Do not disrespect your partner's privacy.* What's fun for the two of you might be somebody else's idea of abuse. Your bedroom should be like Las Vegas: What happens there stays there.

7 • *Feel no shame for your own desires.* Half the people who disapprove of your taste for sexual submission are motivated by envy.

8 • *Do not put yourself down for what you cannot or will not do.* The fact that your partner wants a certain thing from you that isn't on your menu is no reflection on you, but it will certainly be a reflection on that person if he or she tries to force the issue.

Chapter 17

EROTIC SPANKING: NAUGHTY, NAUGHTY, AND OH SO NICE

love the prespanking moments almost as much as I love the spanking itself. Splayed over his lap, legs immodestly open, I relax under his expert touch. He speaks in a soothing tone as he cups my butt cheek and gives it a squeeze, subtly manipulating my pussy. "What a nice ass you have. So inviting." And then, *thwack!* Ooh! I wiggle on his knee. *Umm* . . . and then he's back to the gentle massage. It builds up from there, as he alternates between spanking and fondling until my butt is pink all over and I'm very excited, eager for what's next.

I first became aware of sexy spanking as a flirty thing when my boyfriend of the time smacked my backside spontaneously during a robust round of doggy-style intercourse. We had been going at it hot and heavy, and there was no planning or negotiation involved, which is not a method of discovery I would recommend to others. Luckily, I liked it instantly, and we did it a lot after that. I really enjoyed the force of the blow reverberating through the muscle of my butt. I liked the refreshing sensation of the unexpected impact on my skin. I liked the rush of pure animal vigor and exhilaration. I liked it then, and I like it now. Fortunately, you have access to more information than that available to me at the time.

I was never punitively spanked as a child and had no personal familiarity with erotic-spanking culture. My backside has simply proved an irresistible target to lovers over the years, and the unexpected smack here and there has always produced a reflexive rush of undeniable titillation. I didn't view myself as "kinky" for responding in this way. I just knew that, during on- or offscreen sex, I really, really liked a thump on my rump. Never one to leave an avenue of sexual adventure unexplored, I have subsequently sought out spanking-oriented partners who have initiated me into the more sophisticated delights the practice can afford.

When it comes to erotic spanking, attitudes are rarely neutral. It's a form of pleasure play that needs no explanation to those so inclined and remains essentially inexplicable to those not. For some, it conjures unpleasant associations and/or raises troubling questions. As with any form of sexual experimentation, the first and most important ingredient in creating a satisfying and pleasurable outcome is mutual desire. For obvious reasons, and some less obvious, spanking play requires especially diligent thinking and talking through. Not so much as a single smack to the derriere is permissible without a negotiated agreement. The potential for abuse is inherent in percussive play of any sort, and it should never be attempted unless and until all concerns of both part-

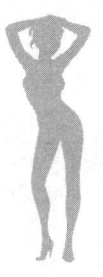

ners have been directly and satisfactorily addressed. There is no middle ground between consensual spanking play and assault.

Why Spank?

The first and most obvious question to address is why? Why would lovers want to spank each other in the first place? Isn't spanking, after all, a rather antiquated form of punishment that liberal-minded societies have, for the most part, relegated to the past? Certainly that is its historical construction. Like those of many seemingly peculiar social behaviors that are otherwise difficult to explain, its roots may lie in desires far removed from its most common applications.

In its erotic use, spanking is decoupled from its social manifestations and reconnected somewhere closer to the source of the impulse that gives rise to the practice. Let me be clear on this point. I don't believe that spanking has any licit purpose outside of sex play between consenting adults, and I regard it under any other circumstances as a veiled form of sexual battery by whomever or however it is employed even outside of an acknowledged sexual context. I entertain nothing but the darkest suspicions regarding the motives of those who advocate it for nonsexual purposes, including child rearing, though that is a discussion for another book.

When sex partners spank, it's not for the "benefit" of one person's education at the expense of another's reluctant labor; it's for the pleasure of both. The primary reason to spank is simple: It feels good! When sexually aroused, the neural receptors in the well-padded tissue of the gluteals process a hard smack as strong, exciting stimulation. Absent a punitive context and the fear of harm at the hands of an authority figure, spanking is a sort of intense caress, producing a temporary sensation of heat at the impact site that, along with a rippling vibration, naturally travels inward toward the genitalia. In purely physiological terms, spanking, short of the threshold of actual pain, belongs in the same category with jalapeño peppers and roller-coaster rides.

The body reacts to the focused intensity of the sensation with a spike in the level of arousal. Undoubtedly, this response gives rise to the "guilty-pleasure" aspect of spanking experiences outside of openly eroticized circumstances. As we'll see, that accompanying psychological charge can also be integrated into a playful, pleasure-oriented scenario, but it isn't required. Many people enjoy erotic spanking at a purely physical level, both giving and receiving, without any of the ritual trappings required by those who practice it as a fetishistic activity.

There is no better or worse in this choice of play style. It's entirely a matter of taste and temperament. For some, as an "exclamation point" during sex, spanking or being spanked just feels right and "natural." For others, the mental component is as important as the physical experience. For most, it's the combination of elements that makes spanking a hot, sexy condiment to the spicy mix of sexuality.

While there are dedicated spanking enthusiasts out there who regard a good "warming" as an end in itself (no pun intended), for the vast majority of casual players, spanking is a form of foreplay, a proverbial slap-and-tickle situation in which preliminaries eventually give way to a greater agenda of hot, satisfying munching, sucking, and fucking, often with a bit of anal play mixed in, as a nicely pinked rump is likely to attract some extra attention. For me, spanking always leads to, and sometimes continues through, sexual intercourse of every sort.

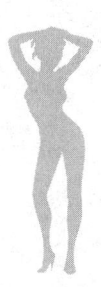

Check the Politics at the Bedroom Door

There has been a general lifting of taboos in the area of consensual power exchange as the phenomenon has become better understood. We now frequently see and hear playful references to erotic spanking in popular music, movies, and even TV sitcom dialogue. There are magazines and contact groups specifically dedicated to the practice, and it has become a common topic of conversation among my workdays audiences. So, if you discover that erotic spanking is something you enjoy, there is an entire social world waiting for you.

Still, no matter how you describe it, corporal punishment (CP) is not PC. It burlesques authority and flirts with physical domination. Certainly, the idea pushes some people's buttons in ways they don't like. Legitimate concerns about the potential for harm in a sexual situation should not be dismissed lightly, but it's useful for any adult to question strongly held negative feelings about a particular sexual act. Upon further examination, he or she may discover that such feelings are based, not upon any personal experience, but rather upon indoctrinated notions of "good" or "bad" forms of sex play.

As depicted in popular culture, spanking play frequently places the female partner in the recipient role, but this doesn't have to be the case, as spanking play is, overall, unrelated to gender identities or power positions in real life. Plenty of guys like being spanked too. In the context of mutual sexual pleasure, spanking carries no symbolic implications. Many men and women feel guilty over their spanking urges, fearing such thoughts mean that they're "violent," that they "have problems" with the other gender, that they "hate" their partners or even themselves. None of this is necessarily true or relevant.

Contrary to pop-psych clichés, not all spanking enthusiasts were victims of abuse. Conversely, some who were abused when younger may still enjoy erotic spanking as consenting adults. Ultimately, somewhere in the space between intimacy and privacy lies the complex mix of the experiences, imaginations, and desires of you and your partner. Judgments based on conjectures about another person's internal processes are not conducive to open, honest, trust-building communication. Why you or your partner like or do not like to spank or be spanked may be a therapeutic issue, but the bedroom is no place to work it out.

Don't make assumptions about the motivations of a partner who proposes such activities, and don't "dump" negative feelings onto your partner when he or she has shown bravery in sharing potentially controversial desires with you. Even if you can't resolve all your shared concerns in one conversation, keep lines of communication open. If, at the end of this dialogue, or at any point in the attempt to act out spanking fantasies, strong reservations remain, "no" still works as a complete sentence.

Spanking play isn't necessarily progressive, i.e., requiring ever more intense applications of force to produce the same result. A spanked body will quickly discover its unique limits. Each couple will eventually reach a level of intensity that's exciting and comfortable and settle there. Nor is spanking play "addictive," superseding other forms of erotic activity. Some couples like to incorporate it frequently in their lovemaking, others only as an occasional diversion.

I have a friend who has been married for nearly thirty years. A while back, he developed an interest in spanking, both giving and receiving, but his wife was not so keen on it. Being monogamous, they must do what they can to please each other, as they have nowhere else to turn to for sexual satisfaction. After much discussion, over several months'

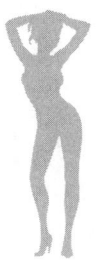

time, she agreed to participate (without begging on his part) about three or four times a month, and he agreed not to expect it more often than that. What made it work was their determination to continue negotiations even when they each got a little scared, he of rejection, she of "having" to do something she wasn't certain she would enjoy.

Context is everything. If your partner is asking for a spanking and you feel like obliging, don't let others' misconceptions rob you of a good time. Women can have difficulty with wanting to be "hit" by their male partners, fearing that it "means" something dark and horrible, while men, rightly sensitized by feminist consciousness raising to the very real harm of domestic abuse, may be afraid of their own "masculine aggression" and reluctant to be their bad selves, even for the short periods their partners want exactly that part of them. If you, as a modern, liberated woman, want to be spanked, that's okay. If you, as a modern, liberated man, want to spank, that's okay, too. And vice versa. No one can tell you what you and your partner have a right to enjoy. Your level of pleasure is your most effective guide. As we've seen, it's hard to argue with a wet pussy or a stiff cock!

Learning the Limits and Making Them Stick

Put simply, spanking is a ritualized form of sexual foreplay that includes, but is not limited to, some striking of designated body parts with hands or with toys adapted for the purpose. The two main components of spanking technique are the physical how-tos and the mental/role-playing dynamics.

On the physical level, spanking is the easiest and often first overtly "kinky" activity couples may attempt. Few sexual initiatives are more fun and flirty than one person shaking his or her ass at another, only to get a swat in return. Even if a person feels uncomfortable with role playing, the physicality of giving or getting a spanking can still be enjoyed.

Before we delve into the psychosexual complexities of corporal eroticism, let's first address the comparatively simple, practical elements of butt whacking for its own sake. The first thing spankers need to understand is that pain thresholds rise with levels of arousal. The more turned on the players are, the more emphatic the spankings are likely to become. That's one reason why it's important to set parameters up front. While advanced spankers may regard bruised behinds as souvenirs and sources of recollected enjoyment, newcomers will be wise to err on the side of caution, if for no reason other than to avoid embarrassing moments at the gym the next day.

In the early stages, spanking exploration is best done under the most comfortable circumstances. The "receiver" can lie across the spanker's lap while he or she sits propped up in bed. Proper placement of pillows helps the "bottom" (to use a bit of role-neutral BDSM terminology for convenience) relax to better concentrate on the new sensations. Stroking, petting, and teasing on the surface of the butt cheeks, accompanied by plenty of genital stimulation from the spanker, or masturbation by the person being spanked, is more than just a necessary prelude. For most erotic spankers, such pleasant distractions are essential to a satisfying experience.

Before the actual swatting commences, concentrate on the different sensations that can be created using fingertips and nails as well as the whole palm. Let yourselves sink into a nice, mutually dreamy headspace. Merely squeezing the ass cheeks firmly feels good to both, and kneading deeply and pulling the cheeks apart is rudely sexy, especially

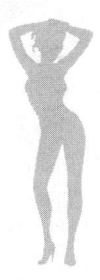

when the anus is stretched to emphasize the naughty vulnerability of the situation.

Gentle shaking of the buttocks can be bootylicious, too. The spanker gets to gaze upon the alluring view, while the recipient feels totally, thrillingly exposed. Keeping the sensual vibe happening, the recipient should be encouraged to grind his or her pelvis against the knee of the spanker or sneak a hand between his or her legs. The spanker can assist in this process as well. At some later point, advanced players may experiment with holding out on such "rewards," but at first, the emphasis should be on raising the heat internally, prior to warming the tail with a firm hand.

By close observation, the spanker will know when it's time to begin, as the receptive partner's body language will signal a state of relaxed readiness. At the right moment, there is nothing inappropriate about either partner suggesting it outright. Start with light taps all up and down the buttocks, from the spot just above the gluteal curve to about halfway down the thighs. *Tap-tap-tap-tap!* Up and down, up and down, all over, taking care to keep to the fleshy spots, missing none. Experiment with different hand positions: cupped, flat, fingers together or spread apart. The flatter the palm, the deeper the impact. Mix stroking with striking for maximum pleasure.

Nervous chatter will soon give way to synchronized breathing and increasing arousal. After a few minutes, both rump and hand will be warmed up, as they first must be to avoid injury to either party. The spanker can use the free hand to pull his or her partner close, creating the sensation of intimacy and safety. It's always a good idea to ask directly before hitting harder. After a few minutes of light swats, the spanker can slow down to a little circular rubbing and ask if the intensity is right or should be ramped up. Don't be surprised if you discover that the giver has less endurance than the receiver when it comes to hand spankings. A well-padded ass absorbs impact much more comfortably than a bony, thin-skinned hand.

Using a cupped hand, the "top" (again employing the BDSM-derived terminology explored in the chapters on sensual domination and submission) delivers a firm, controlled blow to the fleshiest part of the bottom's butt. *Thwack!* The impact, if correct, will make a pleasant, hollow sound, and the bottom should respond positively, with a rocking motion of his or her hips, a squeeze of the p.c. muscles, and/or a pleased verbalization. Gluteal tensing or jerking away suggests that the first swat was too hard or too sudden. Moving too quickly to full-force is a sure sign of clumsiness and/or inexperience. If an admonition from the bottom doesn't produce a quick retreat, it's time to send out for some Chinese food and call it a night.

Should the first solid swat produces a favorable reaction, the top can ask, teasingly, "Would you like it harder?" and so on. Using the bottom's responses as a guide, the top spanks in an unhurried rhythm, varying the speed and intensity to stoke the excitement of the bottom as well as his or her own pleasure. The top can spank toward or away from him- or herself, using up-blows and down-blows, interspersing them with cheek squeezing and anus stretching, or stroking gently with the fingernails. The players can experiment with timing: a whole lot of blows delivered quickly but with each stroke getting harder, slow and methodical thumping, deliberate and distinct smacks, or unpredictable syncopation. Some combination of these elements should be just right. In the trial-and-error process of spanking experimentation, expect errors and address them directly in a good-humored manner.

Spanking play isn't purely physical, as we've already noted. Structured behaviors are an important element in creating the erotic atmosphere. Does the top make the bottom count each spank? Ask for the

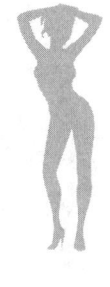

next? Plead for "mercy"? Perhaps there is dialogue between the players, or perhaps the ritual takes place in silence, the only sounds being the impact of hand on butt interspersed with sighs or moans. You'll structure your own spanking scenarios as you learn from experience. Spank for as long as it feels fun and sexy, and then move on to what's next.

The safety issues that arise in spanking play, as with any other sort of percussive stimulation, are significant but not complex. Strike only the muscular tissue of the buttocks and thighs, avoiding the fragile coccyx. Most spanking enthusiasts discover their own "sweet spots" over time, generally in hand's-width hemispheres adjacent to the genitals on both sides. Concentrated attention to these regions will produce the most consistently pleasurable warming effects. To prevent bruising, however, disperse the impacts, whether using a hand or a chosen spanking implement. Swatting in the same space repeatedly will invariably produce broken capillaries. Check in frequently and stop instantly if either player experiences actual discomfort. Remember that, once excited, you may find that your judgment is slightly skewed and that a mildly unpleasant sensation at the peak may produce an annoying, lingering reminder of lack of caution after the fact. Never spank in anger or let emotion get in the way of safety or common sense. And if you're intoxicated to a degree that would cause you to hesitate before picking up the car keys, you just leave that paddle in the drawer.

Costume, Ritual, and Role: The Play's the Thing

For a surprisingly large number of sexual adventurers, spanking—in all its manifestations and with all its attendant stylistic flourishes—is a primary fetish, often practiced with elaborate attention to detail and to the exclusion of other elements commonly associated with sexual power play. Erotic spankers don't necessarily consider themselves part of that "weird, leather-wearing, chain-rattling BDSM crowd." Their tastes tend to be more Anglophile, laced with nostalgia for the snobby, preppy style characterizing the classic CP regimens of the British public school system. In this playful game, strict observance of "social status" and obedience (or the willful lack thereof) to "authority" are elements of subversive fun. So is the fantasy of "illicit pleasure" under the guise of "proper punishment." Costume elements can be major turn-ons, from the severe, high-necked collar on Mistress's dress to the short, plaid skirt and ruffled panties of the penitent "student." Some spanking recipients may prefer high-heeled pumps with stockings; others, saddle shoes and ankle socks. Tight jeans and sneakers work just as well for many. Male spanking bottoms may go for the classic shorts-with-kneesocks-shirt-and-tie approach. The stern "disciplinarian" might wear a dark suit or a school blazer with a crest on the pocket or a sexy version of the headmistress's frock.

In role-driven spanking scenarios, it's often the teacher catching the naughty schoolboy or girl in some forbidden act necessitating punishment that puts the dynamic in motion. The specifics of what's said matter less than the conviction with which scoldings are delivered and professions of innocence and/or remorse offered up. Some bottoms are cheeky and teasing, seducing or goading the top into "doing what is necessary." Others prefer to play the wronged innocent who protests to the end. What's important is that the playacting reflects the fantasies of both players. You write the script together from your combined imaginations. After a few times, you'll figure out what works best and stick with that.

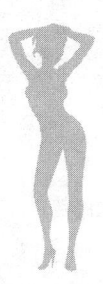

Knowing the Difference Between Punishment and Play

The most important point to keep in mind is that the intent of erotic spanking is pleasurable rather than punitive, even in the context of a "disciplinary" scenario. Keeping the focus on fantasy helps contain the strong emotions that may arise when experimenting with such potent archetypes. As we've seen with sensual domination or submission, spanking role play should never be used as a battlefield for other, unresolved, emotions. If, during a spanking, the mood changes from fun to serious, I recommend that you stop instantly to address the situation and reestablish emotional security. Perhaps a long-suppressed feeling has arisen, surprising both players.

It can be tempting to get angry with a partner for "ruining" the moment, but don't give in to the impulse. The evening's fun can usually be salvaged with a few moments of careful attention to and acceptance of the underlying emotion. When the mood is right once again, simply go back to the moment when both were having fun and start from there. As with all sex play, loving feelings are paramount, so don't go too far afield from them. On very rare occasions the play may have to stop for the night, and that has to be okay, too.

How does a couple get started? Begin by talking, as specifically as possible. Players must decide who spanks and who gets spanked. Some couples switch roles at will, while others never do. Then the context needs structuring. Will there be role play and, if so, what sort? Teacher/student? Cop/speeder? Doctor/patient? Pledge/senior? Perhaps there is no "story" to act out, just sensual pleasure to be derived from the act itself. What about the emotional tone? Is the bottom meant to be sassy, naughty, and "misbehaving" deliberately in order to get what the partner wants, or sorrowful, sniffling, and repentant? Is the top supposed to be stern or loving? The emotional subtext is as powerful and exciting as any of the physical behaviors.

In the beginning, erotic spanking may feel silly and awkward. Keep tweaking the details until you find a formula that's hot for you both, and don't worry about what anyone else is doing. Later, with practice, you will be able to slide into the headspace with just a few cues, but at the beginning, it's good to work out as much as possible in advance.

The most important thing to remember when striking anyone during sex is concentration. Your focus must be on each impact as it happens. Injuries occur when minds are not fully present. Sexual arousal makes concentration challenging, but the two aren't mutually exclusive. Don't think about a few minutes from now or dwell on a few minutes ago. Each spank must be as the first one: deserving of your full attention. No ego here, just respect for what's happening. Also, when using a toy, the top's hand doesn't get sore, so he or she must pay extra attention to the bottom's reactions to prevent injury.

As important as knowing when, where, and how to spank is knowing when to quit. Remember, the ultimate objective is sexual combustion. When naughty playacting gives way to writhing, panting, and

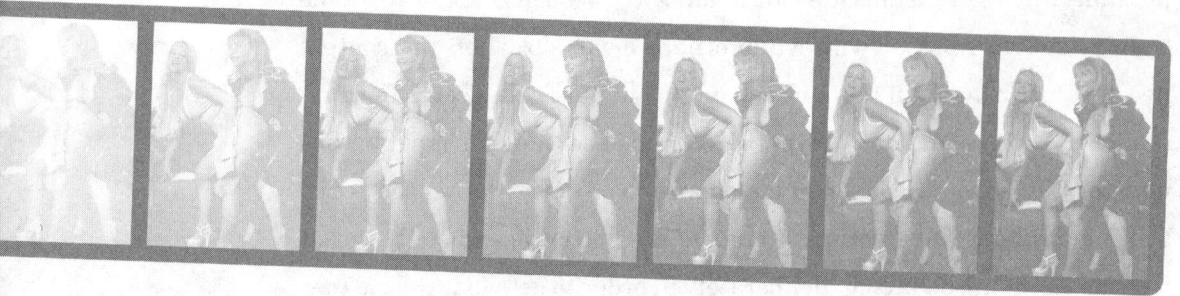

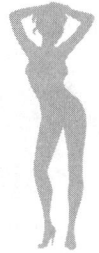

moaning, focus needs to shift from hard hands and red butts to hard cocks and wet pussies. Trust your bodies to let you know when it's time to set the paddle aside and get back to the basics. Spice is nice, but eventually heat needs meat.

Tools of the Trade

CERTAINLY, THE HAND IS THE MOST POPULAR "INSTRUMENT" FOR spanking and will probably be the default implement. However, there are many types of spanking gear available. As always, practice will determine who likes what and in what doses. Some toys will only be used every now and again or only very lightly; others will prove more versatile.

LEATHER GLOVES feel good on both hand and ass. I get extra-tingly when my husband brings out his special pair! I have several pairs myself that only come out for sex play. For me, the sensation of leather on skin is very sexy and makes the occasion feel more special.

PADDED PADDLES come in leather, often with a different texture on each face (fur-covered and plain, studded and smooth). These are good "starters," allowing for an easy warm-up with the less-challenging surface. Rubbing the butt with the furry side feels yummy and sensual, creating suspense for the coming contact of the smooth side. Lightweight paddles stimulate only the surface of the skin, whereas heavier ones resonate throughout the muscle mass.

UNPADDED PADDLES are more challenging. They're quite "stingy" and, if the top is not careful, can leave bruises and welts or even break the skin. It's easy to accidentally go too far with these, so be careful. With hard paddles, it's a matter of taste. Some bottoms love them; others don't.

BELTS can be fun, since they can hit both cheeks at once and have a narrow "footprint" that focuses sensation on a small area. They can also be hard to direct or control, especially for a beginner. You mustn't just "flail away" and think you're doing a good job. Each stroke requires careful aim. The fantasy of a "good whuppin'" must never, ever override close attention to what is actually happening to the recipient.

RIDING CROPS are found in many sex-toy stores. The best ones have wide, flat, leather flaps mounted on stiff but flexible shafts about two feet long, with comfy grips on the other end. These allow the spanker to strike from a distance, perhaps while the bottom is bent over a chair. Crisp wrist action is needed. As soon as the flesh is struck, the wrist should snap back after an audible report from the impact. This will make the strike feel clean and distinct, bouncing properly against the luscious target. Moving the strikes around the butt cheeks soon produces a nice, even, pink glow.

At any toy store, you should be able to test striking devices on your hand or on the behind of your partner. Any good top will test on him- or herself first, so he or she knows just what the bottom is experiencing.

WOODEN SPOONS are very hard and can leave bruises without much effort, making them very challenging and not for beginners. I don't like them, myself. These would be most appropriate in a punishment scenario or for someone with a high tolerance to strong sensation.

The same is true for HAIRBRUSHES. Some tops like to alternate between using the smooth side and stroking the butt with the bristles. As with any hard instrument, some skill is required to make the experience fun. If the bottom prefers a challenging spanking, with lots of complaining and wiggling, a brush might be just the ticket. It's all in what sensation the bottom likes to feel.

CANES are the heavy artillery of spanking. The mere thought of a whippy, smooth, well-varnished length of rattan will set dedicated enthusiasts aquiver with delight, whereas less stalwart spankers will flee the room at the prospect. Caning is the most technical form of spanking and requires considerable finesse, as a slender stick can inflict considerable pain and possibly injury. Practicing on inanimate objects, such as pillows, is a prior must in order to gain accuracy and control. Strokes must be aimed exclusively at the best-upholstered anatomy to avoid deep bruising. Marks are a virtual certainty, so possible public exposure is always a consideration. Very little force

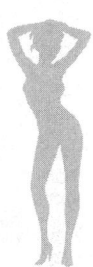

is needed, as the impact is highly concentrated, so always err on the side of caution. And an agreed signal for when the point of diminishing returns has been reached must be established in advance and observed without exception. While "canes" made of Lexan plastic or even aluminum are available from sex-toy shops, nothing bests wood for flexibility and snap.

HOT SWATS AND SWAT NOTS

1 • *Don't rush it.* A good spanking builds from a slow burn to a roaring blaze.

2 • *Expand your target area.* Hitting the same spot over and over will produce an ugly bruise and a bad attitude.

3 • *Find your partner's sweet spot.* A distance of a couple of inches may mean the difference between *ooh* and *ow!*

4 • *Don't forget to reward as well as punish.* A bit of strategic stimulation will increase your partner's appetite for further walloping.

5 • *Know your gear.* Before you strike anyone with anything, try it on yourself to see how it feels and practice on something inanimate until your aim is true.

6 • *If you're role-playing, stay in character but keep it light.* This is all about fun; excess barking spoils the atmosphere.

7 • *Learn to read your partner's signals.* A wiggling butt is usually a good sign. Clenched cheeks and a cringing manner are usually not good signs.

8 • *Vary the mood.* Sometimes a sensual spanking is just the thing. Other times, sterner measures are required. If your partner "accidentally" glues your TV remote to the ceiling, she may be giving you a hint.

9 • *Enough is enough.* Some bottoms like to be spanked and/or caned to tears, but there is always some point of maximum advantage. When your playmate is clearly eager to please, your work is done.

10 • *Never spank in anger.* That's called assault, and if you engage in it, you'll learn a different meaning for the word *corrections.*

Chapter 18

EROTIC BONDAGE:
WHEN TIMES CALL FOR
A LITTLE RESTRAINT

Bondage, like anchovies, is one of those tastes upon which opinions divide starkly and clearly. There are those who can't get enough. There are those who can't run from the idea fast enough. And then there are those—probably a majority—who just don't get the whole idea and can't see what all the fuss is about.

Nevertheless, being physically restrained spices the fantasies of countless men and women. Again, we look to popular culture for clues, and we don't have to look far. From a shirtless Errol Flynn strung up for flogging on the deck of a sailing ship in *Captain Blood* to a sacrificially gowned Naomi Watts staked out as primate bait in *King Kong,* the image of the bound body continues to add a frisson of helplessness to our sexual imaginations.

As the menu of acceptable choices for sexual expression has generally lengthened, I run into more and more couples in my travels who have experimented with playful attempts at boudoir bondage and now incorporate it into their regular love making, if only occasionally. Within that group thrives a subset of eager enthusiasts who invest Captain Blood's treasure in fancy leather gear and go to seminars to learn the intricacies of Japanese-style *shibari* rope work. Obviously, casual adventurers will be more numerous and my own bondage-related observations will be of the greatest use to them, as I don't pretend to *sensei*-level expertise on the subject.

What I do know, from my own experience as both giver and receiver, can be exciting, hot, safe, and fun. For the bound person, or "do-ee," negotiated helplessness provides the opportunity to be lazy and get all the attention (within prearranged limits), with the only requirement being to relax and enjoy what his or her partner ordains. There is also the pleasure of suspense, of imaging all the "might happens" in such a situation. For a person who isn't claustrophobic, consensual bondage in which no real risks are involved engenders an unexpected sense of security as well as vulnerability. My Zen background inclines me to liken it to a state of meditative surrender. Not to depart too far from its roots in the game of domination and submission, however, it's clear enough that the big turn-on of bondage for most of its practitioners is the sensation of helplessness or the contemplation of a partner in the grip of that sensation.

Like other forms of D/s play, erotic bondage can only be practiced safely and ethically within the range of each individual's enthusiastic consent. It's not for everybody. Those who have difficulty letting go of control or taking it may find this form of sexual expression too anxiety-inducing to enjoy. And yet, if they allow themselves to work past their

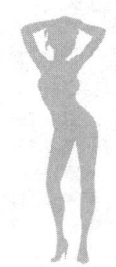

initial resistance, some people with those very issues may find in erotic bondage just the right balance to their everyday concerns. My answer to the question of who should try bondage sex play couldn't be simpler: those who want to and nobody else. If the subject leaves you cold, baffled, or yawning, feel free to skip this chapter. It'll be here later if you ever change your mind.

With the right partner, being physically restrainted can be curiously liberating. It takes a lot of trust to allow another to temporarily remove your agency and then allow that person to tease and stimulate your body to new heights of sexual arousal. To be tied up is to be continuously hugged by the your partner, even when he or she is doing something else to you (like spanking or kissing). However you respond, you come preliberated from all guilt. After all, what your body does isn't your "fault" when it's not under your control. We all like to think of ourselves as free of lingering sexual guilt, but the un-PC fantasies that lurk in even the most enlightened of skulls may come out to play more readily in carefully staged scenarios that temporarily free us from responsibility. Are you sick for having these fantasies? Absolutely not. In fact, there are tens of thousands of people who share your desires, and a lot of them are doing something about them even as you read this paragraph.

For the partner who ties the knots, bondage is a physicalized form of power exchange: Within your prenegotiated boundaries, no one else but you is really in charge here. The visual appeal of the bound person is undeniable. His or her body is there for you to tease and please as you want. This is a power that can be used to positive ends, as your partner's helplessness makes you the source of comfort and pleasure. Bondage games are also creative, using simple skills to enhance sexual excitement for both players. Since it can't be rushed, the process of restraining a person safely creates a relaxed, meditative state that makes the blazing sex to follow all the more intense by contrast.

Bondage taps into primal fantasies of pursuit and capture. This, of course, is the un-PC part. However sanitized by our eager participation, and however secure and loving the circumstances under which we allow it, ultimately, the underlying urges surrounding bondage are all about will: abandoning it or overcoming it. Bondage can be, though by no means always is, a rape-fantasy–associated form of sex play. Some people use bondage play in the context of other D/s activities, whereas for others it is a kink all its own. The operative word here is *fantasy*, and if you really believe that such fantasies are inherently pernicious products of cultural misogyny, I can't imagine how you've made it this far into this book or why you're still reading.

In addition to its erotic fairy-tale associations, there is also a purely physical component to the pleasure of bound sex. It feels good to strain and struggle against unyielding resistance, elevating the pulse, ramping endorphin production, and generally whipping up our cardio as we use dynamic tension to get more excited. And from the opposite perspective, a heaving, sweating, struggling body that remains sexually available regardless is a fine quality ride obtainable no other way. Even the necessity of working around the limitations imposed by restraint, such as the inability to switch positions easily, can be a pleasing rather athletic challenge to the determination of motivated partners.

Ultimately, bondage will or will not excite you, depending on your history, your physiology, and your inner sex life. No one will be able to sell it to you if you don't want it, and nothing will stop you from finding it if you do.

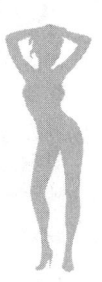

Talk Before You Tie

Okay, so I may have lost count of the times I've talked about consent already, but when it comes to bondage, it's simply impossible to stress the need for it too strongly. Before anything in this realm is attempted, there must be a full discussion covering any insecurities, worries, concerns, physical or emotional limitations, claustrophobia, bad associations from memory, and misconceptions from popular culture, so that they may be addressed and put to rest if they can be (claustrophobia might be a hard limit, for example). If you're charged with running the show, clear all acts first. If you want your partner to wear a gag or blindfold, show your partner what you intend to use before employing it. Eventually, when confidence is fully established, you may both wish to experiment with surprise, like touching an ice cube to a bound and blindfolded partner's tender anatomy, but at first, full disclosure of all plans in advance is the safest and smartest approach.

Likewise, as the person who will be tied up, if there are positions you can't handle because of previous injuries or lingering anxieties, you need to speak up now. It might be pretty to have your hands bound above your head, but if your old shoulder separation won't permit it or if a back injury makes being hog-tied torturous instead of fun, you owe it to yourself and to your partner to reveal these facts in advance. This is not an endurance contest. It's vitally important for you both to understand that bondage is not associated with violence. It's a sensual game between lovers. Do not permit your partner to do things to you that you know will be harmful to your body. If somebody tries to get over with the old "it's supposed to be uncomfortable" dodge, you're in the wrong place and need to get loose and get out of there. Good bondage may be challenging, but it should never be painfully tight or rigid. Bondage should never be a distraction from sexual stimulation, only an enhancement. If a numb foot preoccupies you, you won't give a damn about even the most expert oral sex, so speak up.

Make your rules together and play by them together. Only do bondage with partners you know very well. If you meet potential play-mates through any kind of group social activity, get as many references as you can. It's even better to observe them in action so you can get a feel for their styles. Be choosy. Don't rush into anything. Take as long as you need to find someone fully compatible.

Careful with That Rope, Eugene

After consent, safety is the number-one concern in bondage play. Unlike almost any other activity discussed in this book, bondage carries some degree of inherent physical risk in itself. While ordinarily the risk is not great and significant injuries are few, what hazards there are must be treated with ultimate respect. Done improperly, it's entirely possible (and easier than you think) to damage nerves, joints, and circulation even permanently with a clumsy or inattentive attempt at bondage. The results can include anything from scrapes and abrasions to broken bones and paralysis. These concerns can never be taken lightly.

Numbness is the first sign of nerve or circulation distress and should never be ignored. An expression of distress requires immediate attention. The unbound partner's responsibilities include frequent checks of extremities for signs of trouble: cool or cold, pink or purple hands or numbness anywhere are the body's way of saying "I've had quite enough of this, thank you." In a state of erotic bliss, a bound person might not notice these telltale alerts or might not want to stop or change positions.

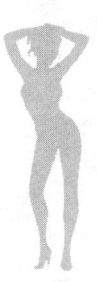

The individual doing the binding must be ever aware of such subtle signals. Of course, any sign of fear or panic is grounds for an immediate halt to the proceedings. Before trying any new bondage technique or position, it's a good idea to watch experienced players do it first, then have them do it to you before showing you how to do it to anybody else.

Always know how to get a person out of bondage fast. One of your first purchases should be paramedic scissors from a medical supply store. The blades will be at a ninety-degree angle to the handle, and the lower one will have a blunt end to avoid cutting skin as you cut rope. If you use locking restraints, know where the key is as well as the backup key and the backup to the backup key. Late-night trips to the locksmith are both embarrassing and expensive. Think a few moves ahead, and you'll spare the both of you a lot of explanations.

Bodies react to restraint unpredictably, even those of experienced bondage players. Fainting, usually preceded by some spacey conversation ("Can I take off my heels?" is a good example), is not unknown when sexual excitation meets physical constriction. Flushed, pale, or clammy skin is also a warning sign. If you observe these signs, get those scissors ready. Be aware that no matter how fast you move, you may still end up lowering a very limp, heavy person to the ground. Bondage play for the evening might just have to be over at that point.

The items you use to attach a human body must be able to bear at least double your combined weights. For beginners, a sturdy bed is the best starting point. Standing bondage looks hot, but overhead attachments are tricky. While there are kits available for hanging bondage hooks over doors, I don't recommend them. It would be a very bad thing for a person to strain, with all of his or her might, only to fall forward without being able to protect him- or herself should the hinges give way. Screwing an eyebolt into a plaster ceiling isn't a good idea, either.

If you're going to get into overhead bondage in a serious way, you'll need long, heavy, forged lifting eyes, sunk deep into roof supports. Test these by tying a sandbag of human weight to a length of rope, belaying it off to your attachment point and dropping it repeatedly to reveal any weaknesses. And make sure the rope is up to the job. A visit to a mountaineering store is a good idea. Welded-link chains and steel cables are even sturdier.

When attaching someone to a piece of furniture, make sure that the backs of knees and elbows are not unduly compressed and that the person can't pitch forward or backward, should struggling be part of the game. Clearly, nothing but a decorative collar can safely circle the neck without creating a choking hazard.

Never leave a bound person alone, even for an instant. If your partner is blindfolded, you can pretend to exit the room to heighten the suspense, but you may not actually do so. A bound person is helpless, and you are responsible for his or her safety and well-being. Know your skill level and stay within it at all times. Have no ego about this; you are only as good as you are honest with yourself about what you do, and do not, know. Your partner's trust must be continually earned. It doesn't matter what you did last time, only what you do *this* time. If you're tying someone up, your attention must be focused at all times on what you're doing. Obviously, significant intoxication and bondage do not mix, whichever end of the rope you're on.

Bondage Basics

Once you start looking around with bondage in mind, you'll find lots of things that can be used to restrain a human body. Some work much better than others. Belts can be good, if they aren't too stiff

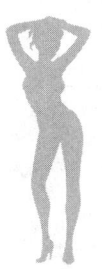

or designed so they might tighten by accident. Cotton clothesline is an excellent choice for beginning bondage. It's cheap, widely available, and not too difficult to cut off if a quick exit is needed. One-quarter- or three-eighths-inch diameters are good: thin enough to be flexible but thick enough to work with easily. Anything thicker will be clumsy to secure. Nylon clothesline is also a choice, but synthetic rope can be slippery, making knots harder to cinch, and can leave burns if drawn across the skin too quickly. Avoid plastic rope, which is stiff and very hard to handle or cut. Be aware that any rope, or even a silk scarf, can slip or tighten when a person moves around. Never wind a rope or strap too tightly around the chest or otherwise compress the rib cage to inhibit breathing.

Scarves and old pantyhose are very popular binding media but need to be handled carefully. The knots they make are very small and hard to undo quickly. They can easily be made too tight. No matter with what you bind a person, you must be able to comfortably slip two fingers between his or her skin and the rope, scarf, or strap. Making bondage looser than that may cause restrained limbs to pull free, which defeats the purpose and could be dangerous, depending on the position. Tighter bondage my restrict circulation or prove impossible to sustain long enough to have any real fun. You do not need to be a sailor or Eagle Scout to have fun with this. A simple hitch and a square knot are all you need to get started. If you find you really like bondage, you can acquire more sophisticated skills as you go along.

Eventually, you may progress to such specialized items as gags, hoods, blindfolds, and head harnesses. These are not one-size-fits-all, so you need to get reliable advice from your vendor. Don't buy on looks alone. Try any new bondage device on the person who will wear it. Some people love hoods, and others hate them with a passion. The only way to know how something feels is to put it on. Gags come in two main types: ball and bit. Ball gags prop the mouth open while, at the same time, filling the space between the teeth. My jaw doesn't allow me to wear even the smallest-diameter ball gag while some of my girlfriends can comfortably accommodate a two-inch version. Bit gags are much more comfortable, and I can wear them easily. Gags of all sorts muffle speech, making the negotiation of hand signals necessary to take the place of safe words, though some of the more clever bondage models I know can speak around all but the most challenging gags. There is always a choking risk associated with obstructing the mouth, so make sure the distress signals are clear before getting started.

As it combines America's two favorite pastimes, shopping and sex, bondage can become an elaborate hobby over time, sort of like skiing. It's easy to drop lots of money on things that don't work or that you don't need. That's why it's important to find a reputable supplier who can and will give good, experienced advice on what works and what doesn't. Buy bondage tackle only from purveyors that cater to enthusiasts, and build up your inventory slowly. The trial-and-error process can prove quite expensive, though with time and practice, you'll come to recognize properly engineered bondage equipment and avoid the flashy but impractical designs cooked up by inventors with little understanding of basic ergonomic principles.

In general, avoid metal cuffs, especially the cheap and cheesy variety commonly sold at sex shops, even if they come padded with fuzzy material. They hurt, cut the skin, and are prone to jamming or tightening unexpectedly. Even regulation police equipment is not a good idea for beginning-level play. Those keys are very small and easily misplaced.

Leather or cloth restraints are available at all price points and in a wide variety of colors and materials. Whenever possible, try before you

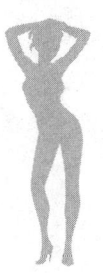

buy. Men and women are very different in size, and no gear is entirely suitable to both. I have man-sized cuffs and collars as well as woman-sized equivalents because you never know who's coming over to play or which role a playmate might choose for the evening. There are also some great bondage designs using Velcro to close the cuffs or attach the bound person to special sheets. I favor these for beginners, even though the full set is a bit pricey. Velcro is very strong, allowing you to apply real tension against the restraints, but it can still be pulled up easily by someone who needs to get out NOW. If you can't quite go the distance and give up all control, Velcro might be just the ticket. As an added plus, with Velcro, positions can be changed quickly and easily, a real benefit over rope, especially for newbies.

My preferred bondage rigging gear consists of best-quality wrist and ankle cuffs, foot-long lengths of chain, and some carabineer clips. This combination is comfortable to wear and easy to use. Keep in mind that bondage doesn't have to be totally restrictive to produce the desired erotic effect. A bit of slack can make for some challenging fun. Attach a foot-long chain between the wrist cuffs, and your partner can still serve you a drink or bring you a desired flogger or paddle. To increase the level of difficulty, you can add a piece of chain between the ankle cuffs to serve as a hobble. When binding someone in a standing position, attach wrists before ankles. Undo in the opposite order: feet first, then wrists. It's easier than you think for a person with bound ankles and unbound wrists to pitch forward, possibly causing injury.

Use that same length of chain to attach wrists behind the back for a different kind of restraint. See how clever he or she can be at servicing you while thus encumbered. Personally, having my hands chained behind my back just naturally makes me want to get down on my knees and suck some dick. You can also lose the chains altogether, attaching the two clips to keep the wrists closer together to render your partner a bit more "helpless."

Bondage can also be symbolic. A slave collar or cuffs without any chains creates a submissive mood without hampering movement. I like the game of "mental bondage," being told what position to take and then holding it until instructed to do otherwise. It's a lovely discipline that makes going from one position to another very easy.

You can also use your body weight to restrain a partner, especially if you both like to wrestle and struggle. If I'm fucking a person doggy style, I will often put both my hands on his or her upper back, forcing him or her into the mattress. Likewise, I find having a person's full mass on me to be very sexy, especially if I'm outweighed by at least fifty pounds. Holding arms behind the back is a form of bondage that feels both rude and intimate. Get behind your partner and wrap your arm around both of his or hers at the elbows and pull them tightly together. This forces out the chest and leaves you with one hand free to caress or fondle at will. I love to sit behind my partner, on the edge of the bed, with his or her legs open (this works best in front of a mirror). I drape my legs over his or her thighs, holding them apart, while restraining his or her arms behind with one of mine. While whispering lewd propositions, I make my partner watch as I stimulate his or her body with a toy or my hand.

Prior Restraint

For some, bondage alone, with a lot of squirming, wiggling, and masturbation is an end in itself, but they're a minority. Bondage, no matter what you may have heard or read, does *not* take the place of conventional sexual activity but rather serves as an enhancement to it.

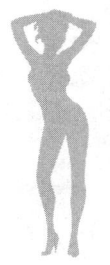

Be practical about this. Don't tie your partner in a way that makes him or her sexually inaccessible, such as legs together, hands behind, and mouth gagged. What can your partner do for you like this? The goal is to make sex challenging, since many bondage enthusiasts like to overcome obstacles, but not to make it impossible, which is merely frustrating. Be sure to allow some room for movement. Tight bondage is good for the teasing part but uncomfortable for intercourse.

When a person is tightly bound, keep in mind that he or she can't self-stimulate. Stop frequently to apply encouragement. Licking, sucking, manual stimulation, buzzing, with a toy, and fucking all serve to keep the energy and interest high. When a person is both bound and blindfolded, teasing with textured things (fur, velvet, leather, fingernails, mouths, tongues, and buzzy things) can be extremely entertaining.

If you're the one being teased and tormented, use breathing and dynamic tension to move the energy around your body. When a spot other than your genitals is stimulated, do your Kegal exercises to keep the energy flowing to your crotch. Synchronize your tensing muscles with your breath holding, releasing both at the same time to maximize the rush and excitement. If you're the person doing the teasing and tormenting, pay close attention to your partner's body cues. The power rush that comes from taking someone to the edge of orgasm and then backing off again and again is delicious! By syncing your stimulation with your partner's breathing in this way, your shared experience is greatly enhanced. You're not reading your partner's mind, though it feels as though you are; you're merely being an astute observer of physiologic cues.

For sexual purposes, keep some part of the bound person's body accessible: mouth, hand, or genitals. If the person is on his or her stomach, make sure his or her head can comfortably turn to one side for breathing. If you want to fuck, say, a woman while she is on her stomach, put a firm pillow under her hips, to help with the angle and the pressure on the small of her back. Keep in mind that the bound person can't easily, or at all, adjust her weight, so you'll have to hold up more of your own.

Until and unless you get advanced guidance from a long-time bondage practitioner, keep life simple and stick to easy, natural, comfortable positions. The most common is spread-eagled on the bed, with a small pillow under the head. This allows for all sorts of bodily torment and teasing. If the bound partner is male, cowgirl fucking is especially easy in this position. A woman bound spread-eagled may need a pillow for her hips to present her pussy for comfortable penetration. Keep in mind that, absent the ability to easily accommodate position changes, she may not have her normal stamina for missionary fucking. Be aware of body mechanics: If a person's hands are bound in back, you can't lie on him or her without causing discomfort or injury. Kneeling postures are excellent for bondage, suggesting a proper attitude of submission and placing the mouth at the perfect height for "oral servitude." Hands can be bound in back or at the upper thighs, leaving a body open and vulnerable to your attentions.

It's also important to know when to lose the bondage entirely.

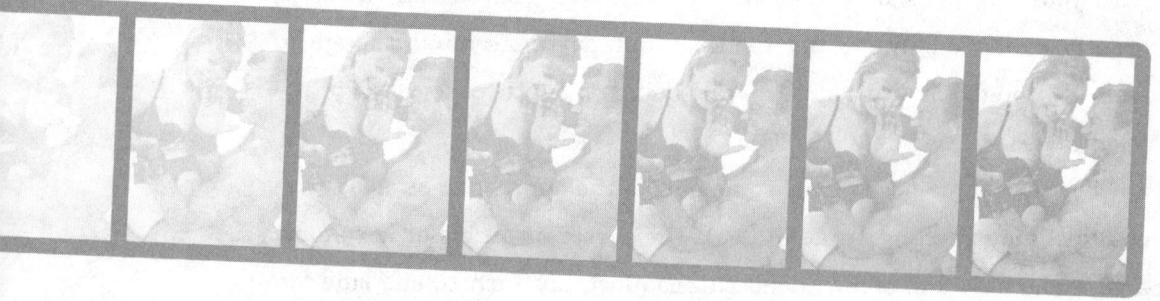

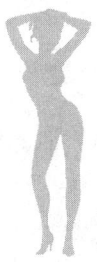

Sooner or later, the bound person will be freed, or very loosely bound, to make full-on intercourse that much easier. But the mood created by earlier sensations of physical restraint will, at best, carry over in the form of an energized atmosphere, like that created by a whirling dynamo cycled to maximum wattage before finally discharging its electricity in a burst of liberated libido. The great thing about bondage is that it feels as good coming off as it feels going on. In that dynamic tension lies its great and durable appeal.

Tied Temptations

1 · *Take it slow.* This is a form of foreplay. The process of restraining is as important as the bondage itself.

2 · *Hold the heat.* Whether you're on the giving or receiving end of the bondage equation, take every opportunity to behave seductively toward your partner.

3 · *Think ahead.* You're creating a work of art together with the ultimate objective of profound erotic satisfaction. Every movement in the process should advance that objective.

4 · *Comfortable is good.* The purpose of bondage is to restrain the body for sexual pleasure, not to inflict irritating distraction.

5 · *Keep it simple.* Excess fumbling and fussing over elaborate details obscure the ultimate goal.

6 · *Know your limitations.* Attempting to impose or maintain a position at the expense of anatomical realities eventually results in frustration and disappointment.

7 · *Sustain the mood.* Bondage between loving partners is all about what feels good and what looks enticing. Every word and

gesture should communicate your mutual desire as in a passionate tango.

8 • *Be ready to move on to other things when the moment is right.* Bondage is the appetizer; sex is the main course.

Bondage Busters

1 • *Don't push it.* If something isn't working right, drop it and move on rather than fanatically attempting to make it happen anyway.

2 • *Never ignore signs of anxiety or physical distress,* even if you or your partner wants to press on anyway. Whatever the problem is, it will only get worse.

3 • *Under no circumstances leave a bound person unattended, however briefly.* If something's going to go wrong, that's just when it will happen.

4 • *No bluffing.* If you make a mistake and something unravels, have a laugh and try again or move on to plan B.

5 • *Do not restrain anyone by the neck, or allow yourself to be restrained in this manner* unless you want to provide future scripts for *CSI.*

6 • *Don't put the welfare of your gear ahead of that of your partner.* If something needs to come off now to prevent a panic attack, use those scissors.

7 • *Just because you saw it on a video or in a magazine doesn't mean you can do it.* Professional bondage riggers spend years learning how to do rope suspensions and other fancy tricks. Until you've been properly instructed, avoid risky, untried techniques.

8 • *Whether you're tying or being tied, never play tough.* You're doing this for mutual enjoyment, not to show who's boss or how much you can take.

AFTERWORD

Unlike many performers, when I entered the adult video industry in 1984, I arrived with an agenda beyond the purely personal. As an exhibitionistic sexual liberationist in her mid-twenties, I was certainly intrigued by the prospect of hot, no-strings-attached erotic encounters with a wide variety of men and women. The idea of making a living by combining two things I loved—sex and performing—was also attractive. But beneath these obvious inducements, I sensed an opportunity for something more subversive. Believing as I always have that total sex is vital to a healthy, well-integrated life, I saw a chance to manifest my philosophy in a dramatically visual form. Instead of merely talking about great sex and all it could do for us, I would demonstrate the principle myself on camera for the world to see.

Of course, my agenda only incidentally overlapped with that of the producers for whom I first shot in the most incidental way. Porn had just gone from film to video at the time, signaling the end of its brief and somewhat overrated "golden age," and, contrary to the nostalgia with which some fans tend to imbue the smut of earlier eras, most of the videos in which I worked were as mindless and undistinguished as the commercial porn of today. Still, I used the industry such as it was to advance my own cause by striving to be as authentic and true to my own sexuality in every performance to the greatest degree the medium would allow. I also stuck by certain core values, including an insistence on doing interracial material at a time when it was considered a risky career move and consistently refusing "victim" roles or characters who used sex destructively or were adversely affected by it.

Through this work, I attained some notoriety, which I used from early on as a platform for espousing my personal beliefs regarding sex and sex work, making myself something of a hero to some and a daughter of Satan to others. My timing couldn't have been better, in some respects, or more perilous. As a matter of both practical and ethical necessity, I became involved in the anticensorship movement the same year I began my video career.

Video had made it possible to view sexually explicit movies safely at home, precipitating an explosive expansion of the audience for such movies among men, women, and couples. This, in turned, fueled a new round of social hysteria, echoing that of a decade earlier, when porn first became legal, with both the religious right and the feminist "left" decrying its effect on society. The issue of porn was sufficiently contentious to cause a rift in the women's movement along the fault line of pro- and anticensorship ideology that persists to this day. The government had its own approach regarding sexually explicit images. Attor-

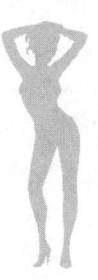

ney General Edwin Meese formed a commission to study the effects of pornography that was so obviously biased that two of its members resigned rather than put their names to the now-infamous and broadly discredited "Meese Report."

My friends, colleagues, and I frequently clashed with pro-censorship forces from both camps at conventions of the National Organization for Women, on radio and television talk shows, and in print. I knew then and recognize now that the bone-deep, highly impassioned differences of opinion on the subject of pornography can never be fully reconciled, but I have a certain inherent optimism that sustains me through long and often frustrating campaigns I believe worthwhile.

Certainly, when it came to greater social acceptance of sexually explicit entertainment made by and for consenting adults, I was fortunate to witness a considerable warming of the social climate. It would have been difficult back then to imagine that pornography and those who make it would enjoy the visibility and acceptance evident in mainstream culture today. Frankly, the notion of writing a book such as this one for a major publisher would have seemed pretty fanciful two decades ago. I don't give myself any particular credit for these developments, which were more likely inevitable by-products of social and political forces already at work than of the efforts of any individual, whether for pornography or against it. I've just benefited by them and done my best to extend those benefits to others.

At the end of the 1980s, the exhausting early rounds of the "culture wars" had left behind two durable legacies: a renewed craving for sexual freedom and détente between the genders, and a woeful lack of reliable information for adults interested in exploring their sexuality. The books were there, but the new medium of sexually explicit video had not yet addressed the wants of consumers who desired literal, explicit, unbiased information on how to have good sex themselves at home with their partners. I found this situation exasperating to say the least. The medium of video blended perfectly with the message I wanted to deliver: You can do this, too, and enjoy it as much as I do. While some sex-education videos for adults had made it to market, they were pretty solemn affairs that tread with tremulous caution when it came to any kind of unconventional sexual expression of the type I yearned to celebrate. In the meantime I continued to make happy, frivolous, disposable pictures in which I played nurses, secretaries, and horny housewives.

Though I had long dreamed of finding a way to combine my skills as an educator with my experience as a performer, the opportunity didn't present itself until 1994. Adam&Eve, a large manufacturer and distributor of adult videos and related products, approached me to do just that. It was to prove a remarkable match. Under the direction of owner and founder Phil Harvey, Adam&Eve has steadfastly pursued a positive approach to the portrayal of adult sexuality and a commitment to progressive social change. It was with the company's resolute encouragement that I created the video series known collectively as *Nina Hartley's Sex Guides,* now in its thirtieth installment with well over half a million videos sold.

It has been enormously exciting to finally share what I know with the viewers at home. Through conventions and personal appearances, I have always enjoyed a high degree of contact with the end users of my commercial products, but I'm particularly grateful for the chance to have provided them with something permanent and useful to have at home. The simple, straightforward format I adopted at the beginning of the series endures. I begin each episode with a detailed discussion of the physiology, anatomy, psychology, and technique of the particular sex practice to be explored. I then perform in a demonstration scene with one or more partners, explaining during the action how the precepts described in theory earlier operate in practice. Finally, I present an idealized fantasy scenario using fellow professionals to illustrate the positive results that are possible from correctly applying the previously outlined techniques.

Topics for the series have presented themselves logically, in harmony with my own continued explorations at the frontiers of consensual sexual experimentation. I started with the basics, things that everyone should know once he or she turns eighteen but is never too old to learn. I wanted not only to teach the physical skills necessary for great sex but to confront the psychosexual aspects of the acts as well. It was by way of the dialectical process of thinking through my own fascinations, dilemmas, and concerns that I came up with the notion of what I call "total sex": a maximization of both the biological and interpersonal potentialities of the erotic experience.

What sets my guides apart from most other adult sex-education materials is that, in addition to supporting passionate monogamy for couples, they're equally, unabashedly positive toward responsible recreational sex, even in its less conventional expressions. Another innovation I bring to what has since become something of a subgenre in the world of adult video is that the person doing the talking is also having the sex. I apply my own experience to the topic du jour and demonstrate how to perform or apply a technique to get the most satisfying effect.

Evidence of the appeal of this approach is certainly to be found in the popularity of the series, but far more satisfying to me is the direct testimony of the many, many men, women, and couples I encounter in my travels who offer their appreciation for the benefits the guide series has brought them. I truly knew I was getting somewhere when I encountered a well-known comedienne backstage at a concert who credited me with keeping her in "several" of her marriages! This, of course, speaks to the inherent limitations of even the most accomplished and enlightened sexual self-realization. In and of itself, even total sex can't solve all problems in all relationships, but it can help motivated partners to enrich their lives together and overcome at least one frequent source of discord and alienation between couples whose other stresses it can actually help relieve.

For those wishing to know more about the video series that inspired this book, all volumes are available from the manufacturer at www.adameve.com. Here is a list of titles to date:

Nina Hartley's Guide to Masturbation

Nina Hartley's Guide to Better Cunnilingus

Nina Hartley's Guide to Better Fellatio

Nina Hartley's Guide to Anal Sex

Nina Hartley's Guide to Swinging

Nina Hartley's Guide to Foreplay

Nina Hartley's Making Love to Men

Nina Hartley's Guide to Making Love to Women

Nina Hartley's Guide to Private Dancing

Nina Hartley's Guide to Sex Toys

Nina Hartley's Advanced Guide to Sex Toys

Nina Hartley's Advanced Guide to Oral Sex

Nina Hartley's Guide to Couples Sexploration

Nina Hartley's Guide to Sensual Domination 1:
    How to Dominate a Man

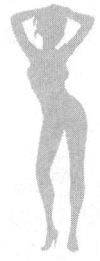

Nina Hartley's Guide to Sensual Domination #2:

    How to Dominate a Woman

Nina Hartley's Guide to Sensual Submission #1:

    How to Submit to a Man

Nina Hartley's Guide to Sensual Submission #2:

    How to Submit to a Woman

Nina Hartley's Guide to Older Women / Younger Men Sex

Nina Hartley's Guide to Older Men / Younger Women Sex

Nina Hartley's Guide to Spanking

Nina Hartley's Guide to Multiple Orgasms

Nina Hartley's Guide to Double Penetration

Nina Hartley's Guide to Threesomes: Two Guys and a Gal

Nina Hartley's Guide to Threesomes: Two Girls and a Guy

Nina Hartley's Guide to G-Spot Sex

Nina Hartley's Guide to Female Ejaculation

Nina Hartley's Guide to Strap-On Sex

Nina Hartley's Guide to Erotic Bondage

Nina Hartley's Guide to Erotic Massage

Nina Hartley's Guide to The Ultimate Sex Party

Looking back, though it took twelve years to accumulate this body of work, it all seems to have gone by in a long weekend. If I've managed to convey some sense of joy and satisfaction to my audience through these labors, it's precisely because I've experienced those emotions (along with plenty of anxiety, fatigue, and frustration to be sure) in the process. And I resolutely refuse to promise not to continue. My fascination with sex and with my own sense of discovery each time I explore some new avenue of its expression remains undimmed, even after what is, incontestably, the longest continuous career of any female performer in adult video. If what I do can be considered a labor of love, it's because I love the labor itself.

Even more satisfying is the awareness of having been a source of knowledge and reassurance to others. My motto is: "I couldn't be there in person so I sent the tape." If a picture is worth a thousand words, then a moving picture is worth ten thousand words, even more when it communicates the subtle nuances of good sex. Video conveys more than mere action. At its best, it also reveals feeling. Done properly it leaps off the screen to ignite the spark of pleasure and intimacy.

I have come forward now in a new medium to disseminate the ideas on which I've based my career as a performer/educator who believes in the healing power of sex at a time when these ideas are once again under attack. If what I have to say seems polemical at times, it's precisely because I understand the resistance my ideas will meet in the current atmosphere. This resistance is nothing new to me. I fought, along with my sisters-in-arms, the same battles two decades back. It's both infuriating and sardonically amusing to find myself once again described as a female chauvinist pig contributing to the pornification of our culture, but it's hardly news. Whether filtered through the slick pseudohipness of fourth-wave antiporn feminists or the junk pseudoscience of the religious right as it attempts to pass itself off as a force for social reform, what comes through, indelibly, is the same stubborn, Calvinist prudery I came to know so well twenty years ago.

Despite concerted efforts to make my cause appear an aberration of a permissive society or an ongoing conspiracy of the patriarchy to keep women in their place through new means, sexual liberation remains a dynamic idea that, once freed, cannot be returned to the bottle. Of one thing I am quite confident: The better we know ourselves through

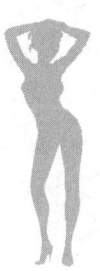

our own sexuality, the freer and happier we will be in all aspects of our lives. I invite each and every one of you to join me on my journey of exploration, to go forward in your search for your authentic sexuality without fear. The best, most relevant book you will ever read on the subject is the one you write yourself, the inner diary of your own experience as a sexual human being. No matter how hard others may try to distract you from the truths you'll find, those truths will remain forever yours to know and enjoy. Be safe. Be kind. Be truthful. You have nothing to fear.

BIBLIOGRAPHY

Anapol, Deborah, Ph.D. *Polyamory: The New Love Without Limits: Secrets of Sustainable Intimate Relationships.* San Rafael: Intinet Resource Center, 1997.

Angier, Natalie. *Woman: An Intimate Geography.* New York: Archer Books, 1999.

Bass, Ellen, and Laura Davis. *The Courage to Heal: A Guide for Women Survivors of Child Sexual Abuse,* 3rd ed. New York: HarperCollins, 1994.

Boston Women's Health Collective. *Our Bodies, Ourselves: A New Edition for a New Era.* New York: Touchstone Books, 2005.

Chia, Mantak, and Douglas Abrams Arava. *The Multi-Orgasmic Man:*

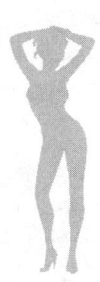

Sexual Secrets That Every Man Should Know. New York: Harper-Collins, 2002.

Cornog, Martha. *The Big Book of Masturbation: From Angst to Zeal.* San Francisco: Down There Press, 2003.

Dodson, Betty, Ph.D. *Sex for One: The Joy of Selfloving.* New York: Three Rivers Press, 1996.

————. *Orgasms for Two: The Joy of Partnersex.* New York: Harmony Books, 2005.

Easton, Dossie, and Catherine A. Liszt. *The Ethical Slut: A Guide to Infinite Sexual Possibilities.* San Francisco: Greenery Press, 1998.

FireFox, LaSara. *Sexy Witch.* Woodbury, Minn.: Llewellyn Publications, 2005.

Gould, Terry. *The Lifestyle: A New Look at the Erotic Rites of Swingers.* Toronto: Vintage Canada. 1999.

Huber, Cheri. *Be the Person You Want to Find: Relationship and Self-Discovery.* Murphys, Calif.: Keep It Simple Books, 1997.

————. *The Depression Book: Depression as an Opportunity for Spiritual Growth.* Murphys, Calif.: Keep It Simple Books, 2004.

————. *There Is Nothing Wrong with You: Going Beyond Self-Hate.* Murphys, Calif.: Keep It Simple Books, 2001.

Kay, Kerwin, and Jill Nagle and Baruch Gould, eds. *Male Lust: Pleasure, Power and Transformation.* New York: Harrington Park Press, 2000.

Lewis, Thomas, M.D., and Fari Amini, M.D., and Richard Lannon, M.D. *A General Theory of Love.* New York: Vintage, 2001.

Maines, Rachel P. *The Technology of Orgasm: "Hysteria," the Vibrator and Women's Sexual Satisfaction."* Baltimore: The John Hopkins University Press, 2001.

Michaels, Mark, A. *The Essence of Tantric Sexuality*. Woodbury, Minn.: Llewellyn Paperback, 2006.

Miller, Philip, and Molly Devon. *Screw the Roses, Send Me the Thorns: The Romance and Sexual Sorcery of Sadomasochism*. Fairfield, Conn.: Mystic Rose Books, 2005.

Moore, Thomas. *The Soul of Sex: Cultivating Life as an Act of Love*. New York: HarperCollins, 1998.

Morin, Jack. *Anal Pleasure and Health: A Guide for Men and Women*, 3rd ed. San Francisco: Down There Press, 1998.

Queen, Carol. *Exhibitionism for the Shy: Dress Up, Show Off and Talk Hot*. San Francisco: Down There Press, 1995.

———. *Real Live Nude Girl: Chronicles of a Sex Positive Culture*. San Francisco: Cleis Press, 2002.

Royalle, Candida. *How to Tell a Naked Man What to Do: Sex Advice from a Woman Who Knows*. New York: Fireside, 2004.

Sprinkle, Ph.D., Annie. *Dr. Sprinkle's Spectacular Sex: Make Over Your Sex Life with One of the World's Great Sex Experts*. New York: Tarcher, 2005.

Sundahl, Deborah. *Female Ejaculation and the G-Spot*. Alameda, Calif.: Hunter House Inc., 2003.

Taormino, Tristan. *The Ultimate Guide to Anal Sex for Women*, 2nd ed. San Francisco: Cleis Press, 2006.

Winks, Cathy, and Anne Semans. *The Good Vibrations Guide to Sex: The Most Complete Sex Manual Ever Written*. San Francisco: Cleis Press, 2002.

INDEX